Infant/Toddler Symptom Checklist:
7 to 9 Months

AF710827

Name______________________________ Date______________

	Never or Sometimes	Most Times	Past
1. Self-Regulation			
A. Is frequently irritable, fussy			
B. Goes easily from whimper to intense cry			
C. Can't calm self effectively by sucking on pacifier, looking at toys, or listening to caregiver			
D. Is unable to wait for food or toy without crying or whining			
E. Must be prepared for change well in advance of event			
F. Demands adult company constantly			
G. Has temper tantrums (severe and frequent)			
H. Amount of time spent calming child during day (circle one): 15-30 minutes 1-2 hours 3 hours +			
2. Sleep			
A. Wakes 3 or more times in the night and is unable to fall back to sleep			
B. Requires extensive help to fall asleep; *specify:* rocking, long walks, stroking hair, car ride, other__________			
3. Eating or Feeding			
Gags or vomits			
4. Dressing, Bathing, Touch			
A. Is distressed by having face or hair washed			
B. Resists being placed in certain positions; for example, stomach or back			
5. Movement			
A. Is in constant movement—rocking, running about, unable to sit still for an activity			
B. Craves swinging and moving upside-down			
6. Listening, Language and Sound			
Is distracted by sounds not normally noticed by average person			
7. Looking and Sight			
A. Is sensitive to bright lights—cries or closes eyes			
B. Becomes excited in crowded, bustling settings such as supermarkets, restaurants			

continued

076-1643753-1

Infant/Toddler Symptom Checklist:
7 to 9 Months (continued)

8. Attachment/Emotional Functioning	Never or Sometimes	Most Times	Past
A. Has difficulty separating from parents, school, or babysitter			
B. Does not respond at all to limits, discipline			
C. Appears anxious or fearful of new people, situations			
D. Needs total control of the environment—"runs the show"			

How concerned are you about the symptoms you have checked above? (Circle one.)

Not concerned Slightly concerned Moderately concerned Very concerned

Comments:

Infant/Toddler Symptom Checklist:
7 to 9 Months

Name______________________________ Date______________

	Never or Sometimes	Most Times	Past
1. Self-Regulation			
A. Is frequently irritable, fussy			
B. Goes easily from whimper to intense cry			
C. Can't calm self effectively by sucking on pacifier, looking at toys, or listening to caregiver			
D. Is unable to wait for food or toy without crying or whining			
E. Must be prepared for change well in advance of event			
F. Demands adult company constantly			
G. Has temper tantrums (severe and frequent)			
H. Amount of time spent calming child during day (circle one): 15-30 minutes 1-2 hours 3 hours +			
2. Sleep			
A. Wakes 3 or more times in the night and is unable to fall back to sleep			
B. Requires extensive help to fall asleep; *specify:* rocking, long walks, stroking hair, car ride, other__________			
3. Eating or Feeding			
Gags or vomits			
4. Dressing, Bathing, Touch			
A. Is distressed by having face or hair washed			
B. Resists being placed in certain positions; for example, stomach or back			
5. Movement			
A. Is in constant movement—rocking, running about, unable to sit still for an activity			
B. Craves swinging and moving upside-down			
6. Listening, Language and Sound			
Is distracted by sounds not normally noticed by average person			
7. Looking and Sight			
A. Is sensitive to bright lights—cries or closes eyes			
B. Becomes excited in crowded, bustling settings such as supermarkets, restaurants			

continued

076-1643753-1

Infant/Toddler Symptom Checklist:
7 to 9 Months (continued)

	Never or Sometimes	Most Times	Past
8. Attachment/Emotional Functioning			
A. Has difficulty separating from parents, school, or babysitter			
B. Does not respond at all to limits, discipline			
C. Appears anxious or fearful of new people, situations			
D. Needs total control of the environment—"runs the show"			

How concerned are you about the symptoms you have checked above? (Circle one.)

Not concerned   Slightly concerned   Moderately concerned   Very concerned

Comments:

Infant/Toddler Symptom Checklist:
7 to 9 Months

Name________________________________ Date______________

	Never or Sometimes	Most Times	Past
1. Self-Regulation			
A. Is frequently irritable, fussy			
B. Goes easily from whimper to intense cry			
C. Can't calm self effectively by sucking on pacifier, looking at toys, or listening to caregiver			
D. Is unable to wait for food or toy without crying or whining			
E. Must be prepared for change well in advance of event			
F. Demands adult company constantly			
G. Has temper tantrums (severe and frequent)			
H. Amount of time spent calming child during day (circle one): 15-30 minutes 1-2 hours 3 hours +			
2. Sleep			
A. Wakes 3 or more times in the night and is unable to fall back to sleep			
B. Requires extensive help to fall asleep; *specify:* rocking, long walks, stroking hair, car ride, other____________			
3. Eating or Feeding			
Gags or vomits			
4. Dressing, Bathing, Touch			
A. Is distressed by having face or hair washed			
B. Resists being placed in certain positions; for example, stomach or back			
5. Movement			
A. Is in constant movement—rocking, running about, unable to sit still for an activity			
B. Craves swinging and moving upside-down			
6. Listening, Language and Sound			
Is distracted by sounds not normally noticed by average person			
7. Looking and Sight			
A. Is sensitive to bright lights—cries or closes eyes			
B. Becomes excited in crowded, bustling settings such as supermarkets, restaurants			

continued

076-1643753-1

Infant/Toddler Symptom Checklist: 7 to 9 Months (continued)

	Never or Sometimes	Most Times	Past
8. Attachment/Emotional Functioning			
A. Has difficulty separating from parents, school, or babysitter			
B. Does not respond at all to limits, discipline			
C. Appears anxious or fearful of new people, situations			
D. Needs total control of the environment—"runs the show"			

How concerned are you about the symptoms you have checked above? (Circle one.)

Not concerned Slightly concerned Moderately concerned Very concerned

Comments:

Infant/Toddler Symptom Checklist:
7 to 9 Months

Name________________________ Date____________

	Never or Sometimes	Most Times	Past
1. Self-Regulation			
A. Is frequently irritable, fussy			
B. Goes easily from whimper to intense cry			
C. Can't calm self effectively by sucking on pacifier, looking at toys, or listening to caregiver			
D. Is unable to wait for food or toy without crying or whining			
E. Must be prepared for change well in advance of event			
F. Demands adult company constantly			
G. Has temper tantrums (severe and frequent)			
H. Amount of time spent calming child during day (circle one): 15-30 minutes 1-2 hours 3 hours +			
2. Sleep			
A. Wakes 3 or more times in the night and is unable to fall back to sleep			
B. Requires extensive help to fall asleep; *specify:* rocking, long walks, stroking hair, car ride, other____________			
3. Eating or Feeding			
Gags or vomits			
4. Dressing, Bathing, Touch			
A. Is distressed by having face or hair washed			
B. Resists being placed in certain positions; for example, stomach or back			
5. Movement			
A. Is in constant movement—rocking, running about, unable to sit still for an activity			
B. Craves swinging and moving upside-down			
6. Listening, Language and Sound			
Is distracted by sounds not normally noticed by average person			
7. Looking and Sight			
A. Is sensitive to bright lights—cries or closes eyes			
B. Becomes excited in crowded, bustling settings such as supermarkets, restaurants			

continued

076-1643753-1

Infant/Toddler Symptom Checklist:
7 to 9 Months (continued)

8. Attachment/Emotional Functioning	Never or Sometimes	Most Times	Past
A. Has difficulty separating from parents, school, or babysitter			
B. Does not respond at all to limits, discipline			
C. Appears anxious or fearful of new people, situations			
D. Needs total control of the environment—"runs the show"			

How concerned are you about the symptoms you have checked above? (Circle one.)

Not concerned   Slightly concerned   Moderately concerned   Very concerned

Comments:

Infant/Toddler Symptom Checklist:
7 to 9 Months

Name________________________________ Date____________

	Never or Sometimes	Most Times	Past
1. Self-Regulation			
A. Is frequently irritable, fussy			
B. Goes easily from whimper to intense cry			
C. Can't calm self effectively by sucking on pacifier, looking at toys, or listening to caregiver			
D. Is unable to wait for food or toy without crying or whining			
E. Must be prepared for change well in advance of event			
F. Demands adult company constantly			
G. Has temper tantrums (severe and frequent)			
H. Amount of time spent calming child during day (circle one): 15-30 minutes 1-2 hours 3 hours +			
2. Sleep			
A. Wakes 3 or more times in the night and is unable to fall back to sleep			
B. Requires extensive help to fall asleep; *specify:* rocking, long walks, stroking hair, car ride, other__________			
3. Eating or Feeding			
Gags or vomits			
4. Dressing, Bathing, Touch			
A. Is distressed by having face or hair washed			
B. Resists being placed in certain positions; for example, stomach or back			
5. Movement			
A. Is in constant movement—rocking, running about, unable to sit still for an activity			
B. Craves swinging and moving upside-down			
6. Listening, Language and Sound			
Is distracted by sounds not normally noticed by average person			
7. Looking and Sight			
A. Is sensitive to bright lights—cries or closes eyes			
B. Becomes excited in crowded, bustling settings such as supermarkets, restaurants			

continued

076-1643753-1

Infant/Toddler Symptom Checklist:
7 to 9 Months (continued)

	Never or Sometimes	Most Times	Past
8. Attachment/Emotional Functioning			
A. Has difficulty separating from parents, school, or babysitter			
B. Does not respond at all to limits, discipline			
C. Appears anxious or fearful of new people, situations			
D. Needs total control of the environment—"runs the show"			

How concerned are you about the symptoms you have checked above? (Circle one.)

Not concerned Slightly concerned Moderately concerned Very concerned

Comments:

Infant/Toddler Symptom Checklist:
7 to 9 Months

Name______________________ Date__________

	Never or Sometimes	Most Times	Past
1. Self-Regulation			
A. Is frequently irritable, fussy			
B. Goes easily from whimper to intense cry			
C. Can't calm self effectively by sucking on pacifier, looking at toys, or listening to caregiver			
D. Is unable to wait for food or toy without crying or whining			
E. Must be prepared for change well in advance of event			
F. Demands adult company constantly			
G. Has temper tantrums (severe and frequent)			
H. Amount of time spent calming child during day (circle one): 15-30 minutes 1-2 hours 3 hours +			
2. Sleep			
A. Wakes 3 or more times in the night and is unable to fall back to sleep			
B. Requires extensive help to fall asleep; *specify:* rocking, long walks, stroking hair, car ride, other__________			
3. Eating or Feeding			
Gags or vomits			
4. Dressing, Bathing, Touch			
A. Is distressed by having face or hair washed			
B. Resists being placed in certain positions; for example, stomach or back			
5. Movement			
A. Is in constant movement—rocking, running about, unable to sit still for an activity			
B. Craves swinging and moving upside-down			
6. Listening, Language and Sound			
Is distracted by sounds not normally noticed by average person			
7. Looking and Sight			
A. Is sensitive to bright lights—cries or closes eyes			
B. Becomes excited in crowded, bustling settings such as supermarkets, restaurants			

continued

Infant/Toddler Symptom Checklist:
7 to 9 Months (continued)

	Never or Sometimes	Most Times	Past
8. Attachment/Emotional Functioning			
A. Has difficulty separating from parents, school, or babysitter			
B. Does not respond at all to limits, discipline			
C. Appears anxious or fearful of new people, situations			
D. Needs total control of the environment—"runs the show"			

How concerned are you about the symptoms you have checked above? (Circle one.)

Not concerned   Slightly concerned   Moderately concerned   Very concerned

Comments:

Infant/Toddler Symptom Checklist:
7 to 9 Months

Name______________________________ Date______________

	Never or Sometimes	Most Times	Past
1. Self-Regulation			
A. Is frequently irritable, fussy			
B. Goes easily from whimper to intense cry			
C. Can't calm self effectively by sucking on pacifier, looking at toys, or listening to caregiver			
D. Is unable to wait for food or toy without crying or whining			
E. Must be prepared for change well in advance of event			
F. Demands adult company constantly			
G. Has temper tantrums (severe and frequent)			
H. Amount of time spent calming child during day (circle one): 15-30 minutes 1-2 hours 3 hours +			
2. Sleep			
A. Wakes 3 or more times in the night and is unable to fall back to sleep			
B. Requires extensive help to fall asleep; *specify:* rocking, long walks, stroking hair, car ride, other____________			
3. Eating or Feeding			
Gags or vomits			
4. Dressing, Bathing, Touch			
A. Is distressed by having face or hair washed			
B. Resists being placed in certain positions; for example, stomach or back			
5. Movement			
A. Is in constant movement—rocking, running about, unable to sit still for an activity			
B. Craves swinging and moving upside-down			
6. Listening, Language and Sound			
Is distracted by sounds not normally noticed by average person			
7. Looking and Sight			
A. Is sensitive to bright lights—cries or closes eyes			
B. Becomes excited in crowded, bustling settings such as supermarkets, restaurants			

continued

076-1643753-1

Infant/Toddler Symptom Checklist: 7 to 9 Months (continued)

	Never or Sometimes	Most Times	Past
8. Attachment/Emotional Functioning			
A. Has difficulty separating from parents, school, or babysitter			
B. Does not respond at all to limits, discipline			
C. Appears anxious or fearful of new people, situations			
D. Needs total control of the environment—"runs the show"			

How concerned are you about the symptoms you have checked above? (Circle one.)

Not concerned   Slightly concerned   Moderately concerned   Very concerned

Comments:

Infant/Toddler Symptom Checklist:
7 to 9 Months

Name__________________________ Date____________

	Never or Sometimes	Most Times	Past
1. Self-Regulation			
A. Is frequently irritable, fussy			
B. Goes easily from whimper to intense cry			
C. Can't calm self effectively by sucking on pacifier, looking at toys, or listening to caregiver			
D. Is unable to wait for food or toy without crying or whining			
E. Must be prepared for change well in advance of event			
F. Demands adult company constantly			
G. Has temper tantrums (severe and frequent)			
H. Amount of time spent calming child during day (circle one): 15-30 minutes 1-2 hours 3 hours +			
2. Sleep			
A. Wakes 3 or more times in the night and is unable to fall back to sleep			
B. Requires extensive help to fall asleep; *specify:* rocking, long walks, stroking hair, car ride, other__________			
3. Eating or Feeding			
Gags or vomits			
4. Dressing, Bathing, Touch			
A. Is distressed by having face or hair washed			
B. Resists being placed in certain positions; for example, stomach or back			
5. Movement			
A. Is in constant movement—rocking, running about, unable to sit still for an activity			
B. Craves swinging and moving upside-down			
6. Listening, Language and Sound			
Is distracted by sounds not normally noticed by average person			
7. Looking and Sight			
A. Is sensitive to bright lights—cries or closes eyes			
B. Becomes excited in crowded, bustling settings such as supermarkets, restaurants			

continued

076-1643753-1

Infant/Toddler Symptom Checklist:
7 to 9 Months (continued)

	Never or Sometimes	Most Times	Past
8. Attachment/Emotional Functioning			
A. Has difficulty separating from parents, school, or babysitter			
B. Does not respond at all to limits, discipline			
C. Appears anxious or fearful of new people, situations			
D. Needs total control of the environment—"runs the show"			

How concerned are you about the symptoms you have checked above? (Circle one.)

Not concerned   Slightly concerned   Moderately concerned   Very concerned

Comments:

Infant/Toddler Symptom Checklist:
7 to 9 Months

Name________________________________ Date____________

	Never or Sometimes	Most Times	Past
1. Self-Regulation			
A. Is frequently irritable, fussy			
B. Goes easily from whimper to intense cry			
C. Can't calm self effectively by sucking on pacifier, looking at toys, or listening to caregiver			
D. Is unable to wait for food or toy without crying or whining			
E. Must be prepared for change well in advance of event			
F. Demands adult company constantly			
G. Has temper tantrums (severe and frequent)			
H. Amount of time spent calming child during day (circle one): 15-30 minutes 1-2 hours 3 hours +			
2. Sleep			
A. Wakes 3 or more times in the night and is unable to fall back to sleep			
B. Requires extensive help to fall asleep; *specify:* rocking, long walks, stroking hair, car ride, other__________			
3. Eating or Feeding			
Gags or vomits			
4. Dressing, Bathing, Touch			
A. Is distressed by having face or hair washed			
B. Resists being placed in certain positions; for example, stomach or back			
5. Movement			
A. Is in constant movement—rocking, running about, unable to sit still for an activity			
B. Craves swinging and moving upside-down			
6. Listening, Language and Sound			
Is distracted by sounds not normally noticed by average person			
7. Looking and Sight			
A. Is sensitive to bright lights—cries or closes eyes			
B. Becomes excited in crowded, bustling settings such as supermarkets, restaurants			

continued

076-1643753-1

Infant/Toddler Symptom Checklist:
7 to 9 Months (continued)

	Never or Sometimes	Most Times	Past
8. Attachment/Emotional Functioning			
A. Has difficulty separating from parents, school, or babysitter			
B. Does not respond at all to limits, discipline			
C. Appears anxious or fearful of new people, situations			
D. Needs total control of the environment—"runs the show"			

How concerned are you about the symptoms you have checked above? (Circle one.)

Not concerned   Slightly concerned   Moderately concerned   Very concerned

Comments:

Infant/Toddler Symptom Checklist:
7 to 9 Months

Name______________________________________ Date______________

	Never or Sometimes	Most Times	Past
1. Self-Regulation			
A. Is frequently irritable, fussy			
B. Goes easily from whimper to intense cry			
C. Can't calm self effectively by sucking on pacifier, looking at toys, or listening to caregiver			
D. Is unable to wait for food or toy without crying or whining			
E. Must be prepared for change well in advance of event			
F. Demands adult company constantly			
G. Has temper tantrums (severe and frequent)			
H. Amount of time spent calming child during day (circle one): 15-30 minutes 1-2 hours 3 hours +			
2. Sleep			
A. Wakes 3 or more times in the night and is unable to fall back to sleep			
B. Requires extensive help to fall asleep; *specify:* rocking, long walks, stroking hair, car ride, other________________			
3. Eating or Feeding			
Gags or vomits			
4. Dressing, Bathing, Touch			
A. Is distressed by having face or hair washed			
B. Resists being placed in certain positions; for example, stomach or back			
5. Movement			
A. Is in constant movement—rocking, running about, unable to sit still for an activity			
B. Craves swinging and moving upside-down			
6. Listening, Language and Sound			
Is distracted by sounds not normally noticed by average person			
7. Looking and Sight			
A. Is sensitive to bright lights—cries or closes eyes			
B. Becomes excited in crowded, bustling settings such as supermarkets, restaurants			

continued

076-1643753-1

Infant/Toddler Symptom Checklist:
7 to 9 Months (continued)

8. Attachment/Emotional Functioning	Never or Sometimes	Most Times	Past
A. Has difficulty separating from parents, school, or babysitter			
B. Does not respond at all to limits, discipline			
C. Appears anxious or fearful of new people, situations			
D. Needs total control of the environment—"runs the show"			

How concerned are you about the symptoms you have checked above? (Circle one.)

Not concerned   Slightly concerned   Moderately concerned   Very concerned

Comments:

Infant/Toddler Symptom Checklist:
7 to 9 Months

Name_______________________ Date__________

	Never or Sometimes	Most Times	Past
1. Self-Regulation			
A. Is frequently irritable, fussy			
B. Goes easily from whimper to intense cry			
C. Can't calm self effectively by sucking on pacifier, looking at toys, or listening to caregiver			
D. Is unable to wait for food or toy without crying or whining			
E. Must be prepared for change well in advance of event			
F. Demands adult company constantly			
G. Has temper tantrums (severe and frequent)			
H. Amount of time spent calming child during day (circle one): 15-30 minutes 1-2 hours 3 hours +			
2. Sleep			
A. Wakes 3 or more times in the night and is unable to fall back to sleep			
B. Requires extensive help to fall asleep; *specify:* rocking, long walks, stroking hair, car ride, other__________			
3. Eating or Feeding			
Gags or vomits			
4. Dressing, Bathing, Touch			
A. Is distressed by having face or hair washed			
B. Resists being placed in certain positions; for example, stomach or back			
5. Movement			
A. Is in constant movement—rocking, running about, unable to sit still for an activity			
B. Craves swinging and moving upside-down			
6. Listening, Language and Sound			
Is distracted by sounds not normally noticed by average person			
7. Looking and Sight			
A. Is sensitive to bright lights—cries or closes eyes			
B. Becomes excited in crowded, bustling settings such as supermarkets, restaurants			

continued

076-1643753-1

Infant/Toddler Symptom Checklist:
7 to 9 Months (continued)

	Never or Sometimes	Most Times	Past
8. Attachment/Emotional Functioning			
A. Has difficulty separating from parents, school, or babysitter			
B. Does not respond at all to limits, discipline			
C. Appears anxious or fearful of new people, situations			
D. Needs total control of the environment—"runs the show"			

How concerned are you about the symptoms you have checked above? (Circle one.)

Not concerned   Slightly concerned   Moderately concerned   Very concerned

Comments:

Infant/Toddler Symptom Checklist:
7 to 9 Months

Name________________________________ Date______________

	Never or Sometimes	Most Times	Past
1. Self-Regulation			
A. Is frequently irritable, fussy			
B. Goes easily from whimper to intense cry			
C. Can't calm self effectively by sucking on pacifier, looking at toys, or listening to caregiver			
D. Is unable to wait for food or toy without crying or whining			
E. Must be prepared for change well in advance of event			
F. Demands adult company constantly			
G. Has temper tantrums (severe and frequent)			
H. Amount of time spent calming child during day (circle one): 15-30 minutes 1-2 hours 3 hours +			
2. Sleep			
A. Wakes 3 or more times in the night and is unable to fall back to sleep			
B. Requires extensive help to fall asleep; *specify:* rocking, long walks, stroking hair, car ride, other____________			
3. Eating or Feeding			
Gags or vomits			
4. Dressing, Bathing, Touch			
A. Is distressed by having face or hair washed			
B. Resists being placed in certain positions; for example, stomach or back			
5. Movement			
A. Is in constant movement—rocking, running about, unable to sit still for an activity			
B. Craves swinging and moving upside-down			
6. Listening, Language and Sound			
Is distracted by sounds not normally noticed by average person			
7. Looking and Sight			
A. Is sensitive to bright lights—cries or closes eyes			
B. Becomes excited in crowded, bustling settings such as supermarkets, restaurants			

continued

076-1643753-1

Infant/Toddler Symptom Checklist:
7 to 9 Months (continued)

	Never or Sometimes	Most Times	Past
8. Attachment/Emotional Functioning			
A. Has difficulty separating from parents, school, or babysitter			
B. Does not respond at all to limits, discipline			
C. Appears anxious or fearful of new people, situations			
D. Needs total control of the environment—"runs the show"			

How concerned are you about the symptoms you have checked above? (Circle one.)

Not concerned   Slightly concerned   Moderately concerned   Very concerned

Comments:

Infant/Toddler Symptom Checklist:
7 to 9 Months

Name__________________________ Date______________

	Never or Sometimes	Most Times	Past
1. Self-Regulation			
A. Is frequently irritable, fussy			
B. Goes easily from whimper to intense cry			
C. Can't calm self effectively by sucking on pacifier, looking at toys, or listening to caregiver			
D. Is unable to wait for food or toy without crying or whining			
E. Must be prepared for change well in advance of event			
F. Demands adult company constantly			
G. Has temper tantrums (severe and frequent)			
H. Amount of time spent calming child during day (circle one): 15-30 minutes 1-2 hours 3 hours +			
2. Sleep			
A. Wakes 3 or more times in the night and is unable to fall back to sleep			
B. Requires extensive help to fall asleep; *specify:* rocking, long walks, stroking hair, car ride, other__________			
3. Eating or Feeding			
Gags or vomits			
4. Dressing, Bathing, Touch			
A. Is distressed by having face or hair washed			
B. Resists being placed in certain positions; for example, stomach or back			
5. Movement			
A. Is in constant movement—rocking, running about, unable to sit still for an activity			
B. Craves swinging and moving upside-down			
6. Listening, Language and Sound			
Is distracted by sounds not normally noticed by average person			
7. Looking and Sight			
A. Is sensitive to bright lights—cries or closes eyes			
B. Becomes excited in crowded, bustling settings such as supermarkets, restaurants			

continued

076-1643753-1

Infant/Toddler Symptom Checklist:
7 to 9 Months (continued)

	Never or Sometimes	Most Times	Past
8. Attachment/Emotional Functioning			
A. Has difficulty separating from parents, school, or babysitter			
B. Does not respond at all to limits, discipline			
C. Appears anxious or fearful of new people, situations			
D. Needs total control of the environment—"runs the show"			

How concerned are you about the symptoms you have checked above? (Circle one.)

Not concerned Slightly concerned Moderately concerned Very concerned

Comments:

Infant/Toddler Symptom Checklist:
7 to 9 Months

Name________________________________ Date______________

	Never or Sometimes	Most Times	Past
1. Self-Regulation			
A. Is frequently irritable, fussy			
B. Goes easily from whimper to intense cry			
C. Can't calm self effectively by sucking on pacifier, looking at toys, or listening to caregiver			
D. Is unable to wait for food or toy without crying or whining			
E. Must be prepared for change well in advance of event			
F. Demands adult company constantly			
G. Has temper tantrums (severe and frequent)			
H. Amount of time spent calming child during day (circle one): 15-30 minutes 1-2 hours 3 hours +			
2. Sleep			
A. Wakes 3 or more times in the night and is unable to fall back to sleep			
B. Requires extensive help to fall asleep; *specify:* rocking, long walks, stroking hair, car ride, other____________			
3. Eating or Feeding			
Gags or vomits			
4. Dressing, Bathing, Touch			
A. Is distressed by having face or hair washed			
B. Resists being placed in certain positions; for example, stomach or back			
5. Movement			
A. Is in constant movement—rocking, running about, unable to sit still for an activity			
B. Craves swinging and moving upside-down			
6. Listening, Language and Sound			
Is distracted by sounds not normally noticed by average person			
7. Looking and Sight			
A. Is sensitive to bright lights—cries or closes eyes			
B. Becomes excited in crowded, bustling settings such as supermarkets, restaurants			

continued

076-1643753-1

Infant/Toddler Symptom Checklist:
7 to 9 Months (continued)

	Never or Sometimes	Most Times	Past
8. Attachment/Emotional Functioning			
A. Has difficulty separating from parents, school, or babysitter			
B. Does not respond at all to limits, discipline			
C. Appears anxious or fearful of new people, situations			
D. Needs total control of the environment—"runs the show"			

How concerned are you about the symptoms you have checked above? (Circle one.)

Not concerned Slightly concerned Moderately concerned Very concerned

Comments:

Infant/Toddler Symptom Checklist:
7 to 9 Months

Name______________________________ Date______________

	Never or Sometimes	Most Times	Past
1. Self-Regulation			
A. Is frequently irritable, fussy			
B. Goes easily from whimper to intense cry			
C. Can't calm self effectively by sucking on pacifier, looking at toys, or listening to caregiver			
D. Is unable to wait for food or toy without crying or whining			
E. Must be prepared for change well in advance of event			
F. Demands adult company constantly			
G. Has temper tantrums (severe and frequent)			
H. Amount of time spent calming child during day (circle one): 15-30 minutes 1-2 hours 3 hours +			
2. Sleep			
A. Wakes 3 or more times in the night and is unable to fall back to sleep			
B. Requires extensive help to fall asleep; *specify:* rocking, long walks, stroking hair, car ride, other____________			
3. Eating or Feeding			
Gags or vomits			
4. Dressing, Bathing, Touch			
A. Is distressed by having face or hair washed			
B. Resists being placed in certain positions; for example, stomach or back			
5. Movement			
A. Is in constant movement—rocking, running about, unable to sit still for an activity			
B. Craves swinging and moving upside-down			
6. Listening, Language and Sound			
Is distracted by sounds not normally noticed by average person			
7. Looking and Sight			
A. Is sensitive to bright lights—cries or closes eyes			
B. Becomes excited in crowded, bustling settings such as supermarkets, restaurants			

continued

076-1643753-1

Infant/Toddler Symptom Checklist: 7 to 9 Months (continued)

8. Attachment/Emotional Functioning	Never or Sometimes	Most Times	Past
A. Has difficulty separating from parents, school, or babysitter			
B. Does not respond at all to limits, discipline			
C. Appears anxious or fearful of new people, situations			
D. Needs total control of the environment—"runs the show"			

How concerned are you about the symptoms you have checked above? (Circle one.)

Not concerned   Slightly concerned   Moderately concerned   Very concerned

Comments:

Infant/Toddler Symptom Checklist:
7 to 9 Months

Name________________________________ Date______________

	Never or Sometimes	Most Times	Past
1. Self-Regulation			
A. Is frequently irritable, fussy			
B. Goes easily from whimper to intense cry			
C. Can't calm self effectively by sucking on pacifier, looking at toys, or listening to caregiver			
D. Is unable to wait for food or toy without crying or whining			
E. Must be prepared for change well in advance of event			
F. Demands adult company constantly			
G. Has temper tantrums (severe and frequent)			
H. Amount of time spent calming child during day (circle one): 15-30 minutes 1-2 hours 3 hours +			
2. Sleep			
A. Wakes 3 or more times in the night and is unable to fall back to sleep			
B. Requires extensive help to fall asleep; *specify:* rocking, long walks, stroking hair, car ride, other__________			
3. Eating or Feeding			
Gags or vomits			
4. Dressing, Bathing, Touch			
A. Is distressed by having face or hair washed			
B. Resists being placed in certain positions; for example, stomach or back			
5. Movement			
A. Is in constant movement—rocking, running about, unable to sit still for an activity			
B. Craves swinging and moving upside-down			
6. Listening, Language and Sound			
Is distracted by sounds not normally noticed by average person			
7. Looking and Sight			
A. Is sensitive to bright lights—cries or closes eyes			
B. Becomes excited in crowded, bustling settings such as supermarkets, restaurants			

continued

076-1643753-1

Infant/Toddler Symptom Checklist: 7 to 9 Months (continued)

	Never or Sometimes	Most Times	Past
8. Attachment/Emotional Functioning			
A. Has difficulty separating from parents, school, or babysitter			
B. Does not respond at all to limits, discipline			
C. Appears anxious or fearful of new people, situations			
D. Needs total control of the environment—"runs the show"			

How concerned are you about the symptoms you have checked above? (Circle one.)

Not concerned   Slightly concerned   Moderately concerned   Very concerned

Comments:

Infant/Toddler Symptom Checklist:
7 to 9 Months

Name______________________________ Date______________

	Never or Sometimes	Most Times	Past
1. Self-Regulation			
A. Is frequently irritable, fussy			
B. Goes easily from whimper to intense cry			
C. Can't calm self effectively by sucking on pacifier, looking at toys, or listening to caregiver			
D. Is unable to wait for food or toy without crying or whining			
E. Must be prepared for change well in advance of event			
F. Demands adult company constantly			
G. Has temper tantrums (severe and frequent)			
H. Amount of time spent calming child during day (circle one): 15-30 minutes 1-2 hours 3 hours +			
2. Sleep			
A. Wakes 3 or more times in the night and is unable to fall back to sleep			
B. Requires extensive help to fall asleep; *specify:* rocking, long walks, stroking hair, car ride, other__________			
3. Eating or Feeding			
Gags or vomits			
4. Dressing, Bathing, Touch			
A. Is distressed by having face or hair washed			
B. Resists being placed in certain positions; for example, stomach or back			
5. Movement			
A. Is in constant movement—rocking, running about, unable to sit still for an activity			
B. Craves swinging and moving upside-down			
6. Listening, Language and Sound			
Is distracted by sounds not normally noticed by average person			
7. Looking and Sight			
A. Is sensitive to bright lights—cries or closes eyes			
B. Becomes excited in crowded, bustling settings such as supermarkets, restaurants			

continued

076-1643753-1

Infant/Toddler Symptom Checklist:
7 to 9 Months (continued)

	Never or Sometimes	Most Times	Past
8. Attachment/Emotional Functioning			
A. Has difficulty separating from parents, school, or babysitter			
B. Does not respond at all to limits, discipline			
C. Appears anxious or fearful of new people, situations			
D. Needs total control of the environment—"runs the show"			

How concerned are you about the symptoms you have checked above? (Circle one.)

Not concerned Slightly concerned Moderately concerned Very concerned

Comments:

Infant/Toddler Symptom Checklist:
7 to 9 Months

Name____________________________________ Date______________

	Never or Sometimes	Most Times	Past
1. Self-Regulation			
A. Is frequently irritable, fussy			
B. Goes easily from whimper to intense cry			
C. Can't calm self effectively by sucking on pacifier, looking at toys, or listening to caregiver			
D. Is unable to wait for food or toy without crying or whining			
E. Must be prepared for change well in advance of event			
F. Demands adult company constantly			
G. Has temper tantrums (severe and frequent)			
H. Amount of time spent calming child during day (circle one): 15-30 minutes 1-2 hours 3 hours +			
2. Sleep			
A. Wakes 3 or more times in the night and is unable to fall back to sleep			
B. Requires extensive help to fall asleep; *specify:* rocking, long walks, stroking hair, car ride, other______________			
3. Eating or Feeding			
Gags or vomits			
4. Dressing, Bathing, Touch			
A. Is distressed by having face or hair washed			
B. Resists being placed in certain positions; for example, stomach or back			
5. Movement			
A. Is in constant movement—rocking, running about, unable to sit still for an activity			
B. Craves swinging and moving upside-down			
6. Listening, Language and Sound			
Is distracted by sounds not normally noticed by average person			
7. Looking and Sight			
A. Is sensitive to bright lights—cries or closes eyes			
B. Becomes excited in crowded, bustling settings such as supermarkets, restaurants			

continued

076-1643753-1

Infant/Toddler Symptom Checklist:
7 to 9 Months (continued)

8. Attachment/Emotional Functioning	Never or Sometimes	Most Times	Past
A. Has difficulty separating from parents, school, or babysitter			
B. Does not respond at all to limits, discipline			
C. Appears anxious or fearful of new people, situations			
D. Needs total control of the environment—"runs the show"			

How concerned are you about the symptoms you have checked above? (Circle one.)

Not concerned   Slightly concerned   Moderately concerned   Very concerned

Comments:

Infant/Toddler Symptom Checklist:
7 to 9 Months

Name______________________________ Date______________

	Never or Sometimes	Most Times	Past
1. Self-Regulation			
A. Is frequently irritable, fussy			
B. Goes easily from whimper to intense cry			
C. Can't calm self effectively by sucking on pacifier, looking at toys, or listening to caregiver			
D. Is unable to wait for food or toy without crying or whining			
E. Must be prepared for change well in advance of event			
F. Demands adult company constantly			
G. Has temper tantrums (severe and frequent)			
H. Amount of time spent calming child during day (circle one): 15-30 minutes 1-2 hours 3 hours +			
2. Sleep			
A. Wakes 3 or more times in the night and is unable to fall back to sleep			
B. Requires extensive help to fall asleep; *specify:* rocking, long walks, stroking hair, car ride, other__________			
3. Eating or Feeding			
Gags or vomits			
4. Dressing, Bathing, Touch			
A. Is distressed by having face or hair washed			
B. Resists being placed in certain positions; for example, stomach or back			
5. Movement			
A. Is in constant movement—rocking, running about, unable to sit still for an activity			
B. Craves swinging and moving upside-down			
6. Listening, Language and Sound			
Is distracted by sounds not normally noticed by average person			
7. Looking and Sight			
A. Is sensitive to bright lights—cries or closes eyes			
B. Becomes excited in crowded, bustling settings such as supermarkets, restaurants			

continued

076-1643753-1

Infant/Toddler Symptom Checklist:
7 to 9 Months (continued)

	Never or Sometimes	Most Times	Past
8. Attachment/Emotional Functioning			
A. Has difficulty separating from parents, school, or babysitter			
B. Does not respond at all to limits, discipline			
C. Appears anxious or fearful of new people, situations			
D. Needs total control of the environment—"runs the show"			

How concerned are you about the symptoms you have checked above? (Circle one.)

Not concerned Slightly concerned Moderately concerned Very concerned

Comments:

Infant/Toddler Symptom Checklist:
7 to 9 Months

Name_________________________________ Date_______________

	Never or Sometimes	Most Times	Past
1. Self-Regulation			
A. Is frequently irritable, fussy			
B. Goes easily from whimper to intense cry			
C. Can't calm self effectively by sucking on pacifier, looking at toys, or listening to caregiver			
D. Is unable to wait for food or toy without crying or whining			
E. Must be prepared for change well in advance of event			
F. Demands adult company constantly			
G. Has temper tantrums (severe and frequent)			
H. Amount of time spent calming child during day (circle one): 15-30 minutes 1-2 hours 3 hours +			
2. Sleep			
A. Wakes 3 or more times in the night and is unable to fall back to sleep			
B. Requires extensive help to fall asleep; *specify:* rocking, long walks, stroking hair, car ride, other____________			
3. Eating or Feeding			
Gags or vomits			
4. Dressing, Bathing, Touch			
A. Is distressed by having face or hair washed			
B. Resists being placed in certain positions; for example, stomach or back			
5. Movement			
A. Is in constant movement—rocking, running about, unable to sit still for an activity			
B. Craves swinging and moving upside-down			
6. Listening, Language and Sound			
Is distracted by sounds not normally noticed by average person			
7. Looking and Sight			
A. Is sensitive to bright lights—cries or closes eyes			
B. Becomes excited in crowded, bustling settings such as supermarkets, restaurants			

continued

076-1643753-1

8. Attachment/Emotional Functioning	Never or Sometimes	Most Times	Past
A. Has difficulty separating from parents, school, or babysitter			
B. Does not respond at all to limits, discipline			
C. Appears anxious or fearful of new people, situations			
D. Needs total control of the environment—"runs the show"			

How concerned are you about the symptoms you have checked above? (Circle one.)

Not concerned Slightly concerned Moderately concerned Very concerned

Comments:

Infant/Toddler Symptom Checklist:
7 to 9 Months

Name________________________________ Date______________

	Never or Sometimes	Most Times	Past
1. Self-Regulation			
A. Is frequently irritable, fussy			
B. Goes easily from whimper to intense cry			
C. Can't calm self effectively by sucking on pacifier, looking at toys, or listening to caregiver			
D. Is unable to wait for food or toy without crying or whining			
E. Must be prepared for change well in advance of event			
F. Demands adult company constantly			
G. Has temper tantrums (severe and frequent)			
H. Amount of time spent calming child during day (circle one): 15-30 minutes 1-2 hours 3 hours +			
2. Sleep			
A. Wakes 3 or more times in the night and is unable to fall back to sleep			
B. Requires extensive help to fall asleep; *specify:* rocking, long walks, stroking hair, car ride, other__________			
3. Eating or Feeding			
Gags or vomits			
4. Dressing, Bathing, Touch			
A. Is distressed by having face or hair washed			
B. Resists being placed in certain positions; for example, stomach or back			
5. Movement			
A. Is in constant movement—rocking, running about, unable to sit still for an activity			
B. Craves swinging and moving upside-down			
6. Listening, Language and Sound			
Is distracted by sounds not normally noticed by average person			
7. Looking and Sight			
A. Is sensitive to bright lights—cries or closes eyes			
B. Becomes excited in crowded, bustling settings such as supermarkets, restaurants			

continued

076-1643753-1

Infant/Toddler Symptom Checklist: 7 to 9 Months (continued)

	Never or Sometimes	Most Times	Past
8. Attachment/Emotional Functioning			
A. Has difficulty separating from parents, school, or babysitter			
B. Does not respond at all to limits, discipline			
C. Appears anxious or fearful of new people, situations			
D. Needs total control of the environment—"runs the show"			

How concerned are you about the symptoms you have checked above? (Circle one.)

Not concerned Slightly concerned Moderately concerned Very concerned

Comments:

Infant/Toddler Symptom Checklist: 7 to 9 Months

Name______________________________ Date____________

	Never or Sometimes	Most Times	Past
1. Self-Regulation			
A. Is frequently irritable, fussy			
B. Goes easily from whimper to intense cry			
C. Can't calm self effectively by sucking on pacifier, looking at toys, or listening to caregiver			
D. Is unable to wait for food or toy without crying or whining			
E. Must be prepared for change well in advance of event			
F. Demands adult company constantly			
G. Has temper tantrums (severe and frequent)			
H. Amount of time spent calming child during day (circle one): 15-30 minutes 1-2 hours 3 hours +			
2. Sleep			
A. Wakes 3 or more times in the night and is unable to fall back to sleep			
B. Requires extensive help to fall asleep; *specify:* rocking, long walks, stroking hair, car ride, other__________			
3. Eating or Feeding			
Gags or vomits			
4. Dressing, Bathing, Touch			
A. Is distressed by having face or hair washed			
B. Resists being placed in certain positions; for example, stomach or back			
5. Movement			
A. Is in constant movement—rocking, running about, unable to sit still for an activity			
B. Craves swinging and moving upside-down			
6. Listening, Language and Sound			
Is distracted by sounds not normally noticed by average person			
7. Looking and Sight			
A. Is sensitive to bright lights—cries or closes eyes			
B. Becomes excited in crowded, bustling settings such as supermarkets, restaurants			

continued

Infant/Toddler Symptom Checklist:
7 to 9 Months (continued)

	Never or Sometimes	Most Times	Past
8. Attachment/Emotional Functioning			
A. Has difficulty separating from parents, school, or babysitter			
B. Does not respond at all to limits, discipline			
C. Appears anxious or fearful of new people, situations			
D. Needs total control of the environment—"runs the show"			

How concerned are you about the symptoms you have checked above? (Circle one.)

Not concerned Slightly concerned Moderately concerned Very concerned

Comments:

Infant/Toddler Symptom Checklist:
7 to 9 Months

Name________________________________ Date______________

	Never or Sometimes	Most Times	Past
1. Self-Regulation			
A. Is frequently irritable, fussy			
B. Goes easily from whimper to intense cry			
C. Can't calm self effectively by sucking on pacifier, looking at toys, or listening to caregiver			
D. Is unable to wait for food or toy without crying or whining			
E. Must be prepared for change well in advance of event			
F. Demands adult company constantly			
G. Has temper tantrums (severe and frequent)			
H. Amount of time spent calming child during day (circle one): 15-30 minutes 1-2 hours 3 hours +			
2. Sleep			
A. Wakes 3 or more times in the night and is unable to fall back to sleep			
B. Requires extensive help to fall asleep; *specify:* rocking, long walks, stroking hair, car ride, other__________________			
3. Eating or Feeding			
Gags or vomits			
4. Dressing, Bathing, Touch			
A. Is distressed by having face or hair washed			
B. Resists being placed in certain positions; for example, stomach or back			
5. Movement			
A. Is in constant movement—rocking, running about, unable to sit still for an activity			
B. Craves swinging and moving upside-down			
6. Listening, Language and Sound			
Is distracted by sounds not normally noticed by average person			
7. Looking and Sight			
A. Is sensitive to bright lights—cries or closes eyes			
B. Becomes excited in crowded, bustling settings such as supermarkets, restaurants			

continued

Infant/Toddler Symptom Checklist:
7 to 9 Months (continued)

	Never or Sometimes	Most Times	Past
8. Attachment/Emotional Functioning			
A. Has difficulty separating from parents, school, or babysitter			
B. Does not respond at all to limits, discipline			
C. Appears anxious or fearful of new people, situations			
D. Needs total control of the environment—"runs the show"			

How concerned are you about the symptoms you have checked above? (Circle one.)

Not concerned Slightly concerned Moderately concerned Very concerned

Comments:

Infant/Toddler Symptom Checklist:
7 to 9 Months

Name________________________ Date__________

	Never or Sometimes	Most Times	Past
1. Self-Regulation			
A. Is frequently irritable, fussy			
B. Goes easily from whimper to intense cry			
C. Can't calm self effectively by sucking on pacifier, looking at toys, or listening to caregiver			
D. Is unable to wait for food or toy without crying or whining			
E. Must be prepared for change well in advance of event			
F. Demands adult company constantly			
G. Has temper tantrums (severe and frequent)			
H. Amount of time spent calming child during day (circle one): 15-30 minutes 1-2 hours 3 hours +			
2. Sleep			
A. Wakes 3 or more times in the night and is unable to fall back to sleep			
B. Requires extensive help to fall asleep; *specify:* rocking, long walks, stroking hair, car ride, other__________			
3. Eating or Feeding			
Gags or vomits			
4. Dressing, Bathing, Touch			
A. Is distressed by having face or hair washed			
B. Resists being placed in certain positions; for example, stomach or back			
5. Movement			
A. Is in constant movement—rocking, running about, unable to sit still for an activity			
B. Craves swinging and moving upside-down			
6. Listening, Language and Sound			
Is distracted by sounds not normally noticed by average person			
7. Looking and Sight			
A. Is sensitive to bright lights—cries or closes eyes			
B. Becomes excited in crowded, bustling settings such as supermarkets, restaurants			

continued

076-1643753-1

Infant/Toddler Symptom Checklist:
7 to 9 Months (continued)

	Never or Sometimes	Most Times	Past
8. Attachment/Emotional Functioning			
A. Has difficulty separating from parents, school, or babysitter			
B. Does not respond at all to limits, discipline			
C. Appears anxious or fearful of new people, situations			
D. Needs total control of the environment—"runs the show"			

How concerned are you about the symptoms you have checked above? (Circle one.)

Not concerned   Slightly concerned   Moderately concerned   Very concerned

Comments:

Infant/Toddler Symptom Checklist:
7 to 9 Months

Name____ Date________________

	Never or Sometimes	Most Times	Past
1. Self-Regulation			
A. Is frequently irritable, fussy			
B. Goes easily from whimper to intense cry			
C. Can't calm self effectively by sucking on pacifier, looking at toys, or listening to caregiver			
D. Is unable to wait for food or toy without crying or whining			
E. Must be prepared for change well in advance of event			
F. Demands adult company constantly			
G. Has temper tantrums (severe and frequent)			
H. Amount of time spent calming child during day (circle one): 15-30 minutes 1-2 hours 3 hours +			
2. Sleep			
A. Wakes 3 or more times in the night and is unable to fall back to sleep			
B. Requires extensive help to fall asleep; *specify:* rocking, long walks, stroking hair, car ride, other____________			
3. Eating or Feeding			
Gags or vomits			
4. Dressing, Bathing, Touch			
A. Is distressed by having face or hair washed			
B. Resists being placed in certain positions; for example, stomach or back			
5. Movement			
A. Is in constant movement—rocking, running about, unable to sit still for an activity			
B. Craves swinging and moving upside-down			
6. Listening, Language and Sound			
Is distracted by sounds not normally noticed by average person			
7. Looking and Sight			
A. Is sensitive to bright lights—cries or closes eyes			
B. Becomes excited in crowded, bustling settings such as supermarkets, restaurants			

continued

076-1643753-1

Infant/Toddler Symptom Checklist:
7 to 9 Months (continued)

	Never or Sometimes	Most Times	Past
8. Attachment/Emotional Functioning			
A. Has difficulty separating from parents, school, or babysitter			
B. Does not respond at all to limits, discipline			
C. Appears anxious or fearful of new people, situations			
D. Needs total control of the environment—"runs the show"			

How concerned are you about the symptoms you have checked above? (Circle one.)

Not concerned   Slightly concerned   Moderately concerned   Very concerned

Comments:

Infant/Toddler Symptom Checklist:
10 to 12 Months

Name________________________ Date______________

	Never or Sometimes	Most Times	Past
1. Self-Regulation			
A. Is frequently irritable, fussy			
B. Goes easily from whimper to intense cry			
C. Is unable to wait for food or toy without crying or whining			
D. Demands adult company constantly			
E. Amount of time spent calming child during day (circle one): 15-30 minutes 1-2 hours 3 hours +			
2. Sleep			
A. Wakes 3 or more times in the night and is unable to fall back to sleep			
B. Requires extensive help to fall asleep; *specify:* rocking, long walks, stroking hair, car ride, other____________			
3. Eating or Feeding			
A. Gags or vomits			
4. Dressing, Bathing, Touch			
A. Resists cuddling, pulls away or arches			
B. Resists being placed in certain positions; for example, stomach or back			
C. Is distressed when clothes are removed			
5. Movement			
Is clumsy—falls, shows poor balance, bumps into things			
6. Listening, Language and Sound			
Is distracted by sounds not normally noticed by average person			
7. Looking and Sight			
Becomes excited in crowded, bustling settings such as supermarkets, restaurants			
8. Attachment/Emotional Functioning			
A. Avoids eye contact, turns away from the human face, prefers objects and toys			
B. Has difficulty separating from parents, school, or babysitter			
C. Appears anxious or fearful of new people, situations			
D. Needs total control of the environment—"runs the show"			

continued

076-1643753-2

Infant/Toddler Symptom Checklist: 10 to 12 Months (continued)

How concerned are you about the symptoms you have checked above? (Circle one.)

Not concerned Slightly concerned Moderately concerned Very concerned

Comments:

Infant/Toddler Symptom Checklist: 10 to 12 Months

Name________________________ Date____________

	Never or Sometimes	Most Times	Past
1. Self-Regulation			
A. Is frequently irritable, fussy			
B. Goes easily from whimper to intense cry			
C. Is unable to wait for food or toy without crying or whining			
D. Demands adult company constantly			
E. Amount of time spent calming child during day (circle one): 15-30 minutes 1-2 hours 3 hours +			
2. Sleep			
A. Wakes 3 or more times in the night and is unable to fall back to sleep			
B. Requires extensive help to fall asleep; *specify:* rocking, long walks, stroking hair, car ride, other__________			
3. Eating or Feeding			
A. Gags or vomits			
4. Dressing, Bathing, Touch			
A. Resists cuddling, pulls away or arches			
B. Resists being placed in certain positions; for example, stomach or back			
C. Is distressed when clothes are removed			
5. Movement			
Is clumsy—falls, shows poor balance, bumps into things			
6. Listening, Language and Sound			
Is distracted by sounds not normally noticed by average person			
7. Looking and Sight			
Becomes excited in crowded, bustling settings such as supermarkets, restaurants			
8. Attachment/Emotional Functioning			
A. Avoids eye contact, turns away from the human face, prefers objects and toys			
B. Has difficulty separating from parents, school, or babysitter			
C. Appears anxious or fearful of new people, situations			
D. Needs total control of the environment—"runs the show"			

continued

076-1643753-2

Infant/Toddler Symptom Checklist:
10 to 12 Months (continued)

How concerned are you about the symptoms you have checked above? (Circle one.)

Not concerned Slightly concerned Moderately concerned Very concerned

---

Comments:

Infant/Toddler Symptom Checklist:
10 to 12 Months

Name______________________________ Date____________

	Never or Sometimes	Most Times	Past
1. Self-Regulation			
A. Is frequently irritable, fussy			
B. Goes easily from whimper to intense cry			
C. Is unable to wait for food or toy without crying or whining			
D. Demands adult company constantly			
E. Amount of time spent calming child during day (circle one): 15-30 minutes 1-2 hours 3 hours +			
2. Sleep			
A. Wakes 3 or more times in the night and is unable to fall back to sleep			
B. Requires extensive help to fall asleep; *specify:* rocking, long walks, stroking hair, car ride, other____________			
3. Eating or Feeding			
A. Gags or vomits			
4. Dressing, Bathing, Touch			
A. Resists cuddling, pulls away or arches			
B. Resists being placed in certain positions; for example, stomach or back			
C. Is distressed when clothes are removed			
5. Movement			
Is clumsy—falls, shows poor balance, bumps into things			
6. Listening, Language and Sound			
Is distracted by sounds not normally noticed by average person			
7. Looking and Sight			
Becomes excited in crowded, bustling settings such as supermarkets, restaurants			
8. Attachment/Emotional Functioning			
A. Avoids eye contact, turns away from the human face, prefers objects and toys			
B. Has difficulty separating from parents, school, or babysitter			
C. Appears anxious or fearful of new people, situations			
D. Needs total control of the environment—"runs the show"			

continued

076-1643753-2

Infant/Toddler Symptom Checklist:
10 to 12 Months (continued)

How concerned are you about the symptoms you have checked above? (Circle one.)

Not concerned   Slightly concerned   Moderately concerned   Very concerned

Comments:

Infant/Toddler Symptom Checklist:
10 to 12 Months

Name________________________________ Date______________

	Never or Sometimes	Most Times	Past
1. Self-Regulation			
A. Is frequently irritable, fussy			
B. Goes easily from whimper to intense cry			
C. Is unable to wait for food or toy without crying or whining			
D. Demands adult company constantly			
E. Amount of time spent calming child during day (circle one): 15-30 minutes 1-2 hours 3 hours +			
2. Sleep			
A. Wakes 3 or more times in the night and is unable to fall back to sleep			
B. Requires extensive help to fall asleep; *specify:* rocking, long walks, stroking hair, car ride, other__________			
3. Eating or Feeding			
A. Gags or vomits			
4. Dressing, Bathing, Touch			
A. Resists cuddling, pulls away or arches			
B. Resists being placed in certain positions; for example, stomach or back			
C. Is distressed when clothes are removed			
5. Movement			
Is clumsy—falls, shows poor balance, bumps into things			
6. Listening, Language and Sound			
Is distracted by sounds not normally noticed by average person			
7. Looking and Sight			
Becomes excited in crowded, bustling settings such as supermarkets, restaurants			
8. Attachment/Emotional Functioning			
A. Avoids eye contact, turns away from the human face, prefers objects and toys			
B. Has difficulty separating from parents, school, or babysitter			
C. Appears anxious or fearful of new people, situations			
D. Needs total control of the environment—"runs the show"			

continued

076-1643753-2

Infant/Toddler Symptom Checklist:
10 to 12 Months (continued)

How concerned are you about the symptoms you have checked above? (Circle one.)

Not concerned   Slightly concerned   Moderately concerned   Very concerned

Comments:

Infant/Toddler Symptom Checklist:
10 to 12 Months

Name______________________________ Date______________

	Never or Sometimes	Most Times	Past
1. Self-Regulation			
A. Is frequently irritable, fussy			
B. Goes easily from whimper to intense cry			
C. Is unable to wait for food or toy without crying or whining			
D. Demands adult company constantly			
E. Amount of time spent calming child during day (circle one): 15-30 minutes 1-2 hours 3 hours +			
2. Sleep			
A. Wakes 3 or more times in the night and is unable to fall back to sleep			
B. Requires extensive help to fall asleep; *specify:* rocking, long walks, stroking hair, car ride, other__________			
3. Eating or Feeding			
A. Gags or vomits			
4. Dressing, Bathing, Touch			
A. Resists cuddling, pulls away or arches			
B. Resists being placed in certain positions; for example, stomach or back			
C. Is distressed when clothes are removed			
5. Movement			
Is clumsy—falls, shows poor balance, bumps into things			
6. Listening, Language and Sound			
Is distracted by sounds not normally noticed by average person			
7. Looking and Sight			
Becomes excited in crowded, bustling settings such as supermarkets, restaurants			
8. Attachment/Emotional Functioning			
A. Avoids eye contact, turns away from the human face, prefers objects and toys			
B. Has difficulty separating from parents, school, or babysitter			
C. Appears anxious or fearful of new people, situations			
D. Needs total control of the environment—"runs the show"			

continued

076-1643753-2

Infant/Toddler Symptom Checklist:
10 to 12 Months (continued)

How concerned are you about the symptoms you have checked above? (Circle one.)

Not concerned　　Slightly concerned　　Moderately concerned　　Very concerned

Comments:

Infant/Toddler Symptom Checklist: 10 to 12 Months

Name______________________________ Date______________

	Never or Sometimes	Most Times	Past
1. Self-Regulation			
A. Is frequently irritable, fussy			
B. Goes easily from whimper to intense cry			
C. Is unable to wait for food or toy without crying or whining			
D. Demands adult company constantly			
E. Amount of time spent calming child during day (circle one): 15-30 minutes 1-2 hours 3 hours +			
2. Sleep			
A. Wakes 3 or more times in the night and is unable to fall back to sleep			
B. Requires extensive help to fall asleep; *specify:* rocking, long walks, stroking hair, car ride, other__________			
3. Eating or Feeding			
A. Gags or vomits			
4. Dressing, Bathing, Touch			
A. Resists cuddling, pulls away or arches			
B. Resists being placed in certain positions; for example, stomach or back			
C. Is distressed when clothes are removed			
5. Movement			
Is clumsy—falls, shows poor balance, bumps into things			
6. Listening, Language and Sound			
Is distracted by sounds not normally noticed by average person			
7. Looking and Sight			
Becomes excited in crowded, bustling settings such as supermarkets, restaurants			
8. Attachment/Emotional Functioning			
A. Avoids eye contact, turns away from the human face, prefers objects and toys			
B. Has difficulty separating from parents, school, or babysitter			
C. Appears anxious or fearful of new people, situations			
D. Needs total control of the environment—"runs the show"			

continued

076-1643753-2

Infant/Toddler Symptom Checklist:
10 to 12 Months (continued)

How concerned are you about the symptoms you have checked above? (Circle one.)

Not concerned   Slightly concerned   Moderately concerned   Very concerned

Comments:

Infant/Toddler Symptom Checklist: 10 to 12 Months

Name________________________________ Date______________

	Never or Sometimes	Most Times	Past
1. Self-Regulation			
A. Is frequently irritable, fussy			
B. Goes easily from whimper to intense cry			
C. Is unable to wait for food or toy without crying or whining			
D. Demands adult company constantly			
E. Amount of time spent calming child during day (circle one): 15-30 minutes 1-2 hours 3 hours +			
2. Sleep			
A. Wakes 3 or more times in the night and is unable to fall back to sleep			
B. Requires extensive help to fall asleep; *specify:* rocking, long walks, stroking hair, car ride, other____________			
3. Eating or Feeding			
A. Gags or vomits			
4. Dressing, Bathing, Touch			
A. Resists cuddling, pulls away or arches			
B. Resists being placed in certain positions; for example, stomach or back			
C. Is distressed when clothes are removed			
5. Movement			
Is clumsy—falls, shows poor balance, bumps into things			
6. Listening, Language and Sound			
Is distracted by sounds not normally noticed by average person			
7. Looking and Sight			
Becomes excited in crowded, bustling settings such as supermarkets, restaurants			
8. Attachment/Emotional Functioning			
A. Avoids eye contact, turns away from the human face, prefers objects and toys			
B. Has difficulty separating from parents, school, or babysitter			
C. Appears anxious or fearful of new people, situations			
D. Needs total control of the environment—"runs the show"			

continued

076-1643753-2

Infant/Toddler Symptom Checklist:
10 to 12 Months (continued)

How concerned are you about the symptoms you have checked above? (Circle one.)

Not concerned   Slightly concerned   Moderately concerned   Very concerned

Comments:

Infant/Toddler Symptom Checklist: 10 to 12 Months

Name_______________________________________ Date_______________

	Never or Sometimes	Most Times	Past
1. Self-Regulation			
A. Is frequently irritable, fussy			
B. Goes easily from whimper to intense cry			
C. Is unable to wait for food or toy without crying or whining			
D. Demands adult company constantly			
E. Amount of time spent calming child during day (circle one): 15-30 minutes 1-2 hours 3 hours +			
2. Sleep			
A. Wakes 3 or more times in the night and is unable to fall back to sleep			
B. Requires extensive help to fall asleep; *specify:* rocking, long walks, stroking hair, car ride, other____________			
3. Eating or Feeding			
A. Gags or vomits			
4. Dressing, Bathing, Touch			
A. Resists cuddling, pulls away or arches			
B. Resists being placed in certain positions; for example, stomach or back			
C. Is distressed when clothes are removed			
5. Movement			
Is clumsy—falls, shows poor balance, bumps into things			
6. Listening, Language and Sound			
Is distracted by sounds not normally noticed by average person			
7. Looking and Sight			
Becomes excited in crowded, bustling settings such as supermarkets, restaurants			
8. Attachment/Emotional Functioning			
A. Avoids eye contact, turns away from the human face, prefers objects and toys			
B. Has difficulty separating from parents, school, or babysitter			
C. Appears anxious or fearful of new people, situations			
D. Needs total control of the environment—"runs the show"			

continued

076-1643753-2

Infant/Toddler Symptom Checklist:
10 to 12 Months (continued)

How concerned are you about the symptoms you have checked above? (Circle one.)

Not concerned   Slightly concerned   Moderately concerned   Very concerned

Comments:

Infant/Toddler Symptom Checklist:
10 to 12 Months

Name______________________________ Date______________

	Never or Sometimes	Most Times	Past
1. Self-Regulation			
A. Is frequently irritable, fussy			
B. Goes easily from whimper to intense cry			
C. Is unable to wait for food or toy without crying or whining			
D. Demands adult company constantly			
E. Amount of time spent calming child during day (circle one): 15-30 minutes 1-2 hours 3 hours +			
2. Sleep			
A. Wakes 3 or more times in the night and is unable to fall back to sleep			
B. Requires extensive help to fall asleep; *specify:* rocking, long walks, stroking hair, car ride, other__________			
3. Eating or Feeding			
A. Gags or vomits			
4. Dressing, Bathing, Touch			
A. Resists cuddling, pulls away or arches			
B. Resists being placed in certain positions; for example, stomach or back			
C. Is distressed when clothes are removed			
5. Movement			
Is clumsy—falls, shows poor balance, bumps into things			
6. Listening, Language and Sound			
Is distracted by sounds not normally noticed by average person			
7. Looking and Sight			
Becomes excited in crowded, bustling settings such as supermarkets, restaurants			
8. Attachment/Emotional Functioning			
A. Avoids eye contact, turns away from the human face, prefers objects and toys			
B. Has difficulty separating from parents, school, or babysitter			
C. Appears anxious or fearful of new people, situations			
D. Needs total control of the environment—"runs the show"			

continued

076-1643753-2

Infant/Toddler Symptom Checklist:
10 to 12 Months (continued)

How concerned are you about the symptoms you have checked above? (Circle one.)

Not concerned Slightly concerned Moderately concerned Very concerned

Comments:

Infant/Toddler Symptom Checklist: 10 to 12 Months

Name________________________________ Date____________

	Never or Sometimes	Most Times	Past
1. Self-Regulation			
A. Is frequently irritable, fussy			
B. Goes easily from whimper to intense cry			
C. Is unable to wait for food or toy without crying or whining			
D. Demands adult company constantly			
E. Amount of time spent calming child during day (circle one): 15-30 minutes 1-2 hours 3 hours +			
2. Sleep			
A. Wakes 3 or more times in the night and is unable to fall back to sleep			
B. Requires extensive help to fall asleep; *specify:* rocking, long walks, stroking hair, car ride, other__________			
3. Eating or Feeding			
A. Gags or vomits			
4. Dressing, Bathing, Touch			
A. Resists cuddling, pulls away or arches			
B. Resists being placed in certain positions; for example, stomach or back			
C. Is distressed when clothes are removed			
5. Movement			
Is clumsy—falls, shows poor balance, bumps into things			
6. Listening, Language and Sound			
Is distracted by sounds not normally noticed by average person			
7. Looking and Sight			
Becomes excited in crowded, bustling settings such as supermarkets, restaurants			
8. Attachment/Emotional Functioning			
A. Avoids eye contact, turns away from the human face, prefers objects and toys			
B. Has difficulty separating from parents, school, or babysitter			
C. Appears anxious or fearful of new people, situations			
D. Needs total control of the environment—"runs the show"			

continued

Infant/Toddler Symptom Checklist:
10 to 12 Months (continued)

How concerned are you about the symptoms you have checked above? (Circle one.)

Not concerned   Slightly concerned   Moderately concerned   Very concerned

Comments:

Infant/Toddler Symptom Checklist:
10 to 12 Months

Name______________________________ Date______________

	Never or Sometimes	Most Times	Past
1. Self-Regulation			
A. Is frequently irritable, fussy			
B. Goes easily from whimper to intense cry			
C. Is unable to wait for food or toy without crying or whining			
D. Demands adult company constantly			
E. Amount of time spent calming child during day (circle one): 15-30 minutes 1-2 hours 3 hours +			
2. Sleep			
A. Wakes 3 or more times in the night and is unable to fall back to sleep			
B. Requires extensive help to fall asleep; *specify:* rocking, long walks, stroking hair, car ride, other__________			
3. Eating or Feeding			
A. Gags or vomits			
4. Dressing, Bathing, Touch			
A. Resists cuddling, pulls away or arches			
B. Resists being placed in certain positions; for example, stomach or back			
C. Is distressed when clothes are removed			
5. Movement			
Is clumsy—falls, shows poor balance, bumps into things			
6. Listening, Language and Sound			
Is distracted by sounds not normally noticed by average person			
7. Looking and Sight			
Becomes excited in crowded, bustling settings such as supermarkets, restaurants			
8. Attachment/Emotional Functioning			
A. Avoids eye contact, turns away from the human face, prefers objects and toys			
B. Has difficulty separating from parents, school, or babysitter			
C. Appears anxious or fearful of new people, situations			
D. Needs total control of the environment—"runs the show"			

continued

076-1643753-2

Infant/Toddler Symptom Checklist:
10 to 12 Months (continued)

How concerned are you about the symptoms you have checked above? (Circle one.)

Not concerned   Slightly concerned   Moderately concerned   Very concerned

Comments:

Infant/Toddler Symptom Checklist:
10 to 12 Months

Name______________________________ Date______________

	Never or Sometimes	Most Times	Past
1. Self-Regulation			
A. Is frequently irritable, fussy			
B. Goes easily from whimper to intense cry			
C. Is unable to wait for food or toy without crying or whining			
D. Demands adult company constantly			
E. Amount of time spent calming child during day (circle one): 15-30 minutes 1-2 hours 3 hours +			
2. Sleep			
A. Wakes 3 or more times in the night and is unable to fall back to sleep			
B. Requires extensive help to fall asleep; *specify:* rocking, long walks, stroking hair, car ride, other____________			
3. Eating or Feeding			
A. Gags or vomits			
4. Dressing, Bathing, Touch			
A. Resists cuddling, pulls away or arches			
B. Resists being placed in certain positions; for example, stomach or back			
C. Is distressed when clothes are removed			
5. Movement			
Is clumsy—falls, shows poor balance, bumps into things			
6. Listening, Language and Sound			
Is distracted by sounds not normally noticed by average person			
7. Looking and Sight			
Becomes excited in crowded, bustling settings such as supermarkets, restaurants			
8. Attachment/Emotional Functioning			
A. Avoids eye contact, turns away from the human face, prefers objects and toys			
B. Has difficulty separating from parents, school, or babysitter			
C. Appears anxious or fearful of new people, situations			
D. Needs total control of the environment—"runs the show"			

continued

076-1643753-2

How concerned are you about the symptoms you have checked above? (Circle one.)

Not concerned Slightly concerned Moderately concerned Very concerned

Comments:

Infant/Toddler Symptom Checklist: 10 to 12 Months

Name______________________________ Date______________

	Never or Sometimes	Most Times	Past
1. Self-Regulation			
A. Is frequently irritable, fussy			
B. Goes easily from whimper to intense cry			
C. Is unable to wait for food or toy without crying or whining			
D. Demands adult company constantly			
E. Amount of time spent calming child during day (circle one): 15-30 minutes 1-2 hours 3 hours +			
2. Sleep			
A. Wakes 3 or more times in the night and is unable to fall back to sleep			
B. Requires extensive help to fall asleep; *specify:* rocking, long walks, stroking hair, car ride, other__________			
3. Eating or Feeding			
A. Gags or vomits			
4. Dressing, Bathing, Touch			
A. Resists cuddling, pulls away or arches			
B. Resists being placed in certain positions; for example, stomach or back			
C. Is distressed when clothes are removed			
5. Movement			
Is clumsy—falls, shows poor balance, bumps into things			
6. Listening, Language and Sound			
Is distracted by sounds not normally noticed by average person			
7. Looking and Sight			
Becomes excited in crowded, bustling settings such as supermarkets, restaurants			
8. Attachment/Emotional Functioning			
A. Avoids eye contact, turns away from the human face, prefers objects and toys			
B. Has difficulty separating from parents, school, or babysitter			
C. Appears anxious or fearful of new people, situations			
D. Needs total control of the environment—"runs the show"			

continued

076-1643753-2

Infant/Toddler Symptom Checklist:
10 to 12 Months (continued)

How concerned are you about the symptoms you have checked above? (Circle one.)

Not concerned   Slightly concerned   Moderately concerned   Very concerned

---

Comments:

Infant/Toddler Symptom Checklist:
10 to 12 Months

Name________________________________ Date______________

	Never or Sometimes	Most Times	Past
1. Self-Regulation			
A. Is frequently irritable, fussy			
B. Goes easily from whimper to intense cry			
C. Is unable to wait for food or toy without crying or whining			
D. Demands adult company constantly			
E. Amount of time spent calming child during day (circle one): 15-30 minutes 1-2 hours 3 hours +			
2. Sleep			
A. Wakes 3 or more times in the night and is unable to fall back to sleep			
B. Requires extensive help to fall asleep; *specify:* rocking, long walks, stroking hair, car ride, other____________			
3. Eating or Feeding			
A. Gags or vomits			
4. Dressing, Bathing, Touch			
A. Resists cuddling, pulls away or arches			
B. Resists being placed in certain positions; for example, stomach or back			
C. Is distressed when clothes are removed			
5. Movement			
Is clumsy—falls, shows poor balance, bumps into things			
6. Listening, Language and Sound			
Is distracted by sounds not normally noticed by average person			
7. Looking and Sight			
Becomes excited in crowded, bustling settings such as supermarkets, restaurants			
8. Attachment/Emotional Functioning			
A. Avoids eye contact, turns away from the human face, prefers objects and toys			
B. Has difficulty separating from parents, school, or babysitter			
C. Appears anxious or fearful of new people, situations			
D. Needs total control of the environment—"runs the show"			

continued

076-1643753-2

Infant/Toddler Symptom Checklist:
10 to 12 Months (continued)

How concerned are you about the symptoms you have checked above? (Circle one.)

Not concerned   Slightly concerned   Moderately concerned   Very concerned

---

Comments:

Infant/Toddler Symptom Checklist:
10 to 12 Months

Name______________________________ Date______________

	Never or Sometimes	Most Times	Past
1. Self-Regulation			
A. Is frequently irritable, fussy			
B. Goes easily from whimper to intense cry			
C. Is unable to wait for food or toy without crying or whining			
D. Demands adult company constantly			
E. Amount of time spent calming child during day (circle one): 15-30 minutes 1-2 hours 3 hours +			
2. Sleep			
A. Wakes 3 or more times in the night and is unable to fall back to sleep			
B. Requires extensive help to fall asleep; *specify:* rocking, long walks, stroking hair, car ride, other__________			
3. Eating or Feeding			
A. Gags or vomits			
4. Dressing, Bathing, Touch			
A. Resists cuddling, pulls away or arches			
B. Resists being placed in certain positions; for example, stomach or back			
C. Is distressed when clothes are removed			
5. Movement			
Is clumsy—falls, shows poor balance, bumps into things			
6. Listening, Language and Sound			
Is distracted by sounds not normally noticed by average person			
7. Looking and Sight			
Becomes excited in crowded, bustling settings such as supermarkets, restaurants			
8. Attachment/Emotional Functioning			
A. Avoids eye contact, turns away from the human face, prefers objects and toys			
B. Has difficulty separating from parents, school, or babysitter			
C. Appears anxious or fearful of new people, situations			
D. Needs total control of the environment—"runs the show"			

continued

076-1643753-2

Infant/Toddler Symptom Checklist:
10 to 12 Months (continued)

How concerned are you about the symptoms you have checked above? (Circle one.)

Not concerned   Slightly concerned   Moderately concerned   Very concerned

Comments:

Infant/Toddler Symptom Checklist: 10 to 12 Months

Name________________________________ Date______________

	Never or Sometimes	Most Times	Past
1. Self-Regulation			
A. Is frequently irritable, fussy			
B. Goes easily from whimper to intense cry			
C. Is unable to wait for food or toy without crying or whining			
D. Demands adult company constantly			
E. Amount of time spent calming child during day (circle one): 15-30 minutes 1-2 hours 3 hours +			
2. Sleep			
A. Wakes 3 or more times in the night and is unable to fall back to sleep			
B. Requires extensive help to fall asleep; *specify:* rocking, long walks, stroking hair, car ride, other__________			
3. Eating or Feeding			
A. Gags or vomits			
4. Dressing, Bathing, Touch			
A. Resists cuddling, pulls away or arches			
B. Resists being placed in certain positions; for example, stomach or back			
C. Is distressed when clothes are removed			
5. Movement			
Is clumsy—falls, shows poor balance, bumps into things			
6. Listening, Language and Sound			
Is distracted by sounds not normally noticed by average person			
7. Looking and Sight			
Becomes excited in crowded, bustling settings such as supermarkets, restaurants			
8. Attachment/Emotional Functioning			
A. Avoids eye contact, turns away from the human face, prefers objects and toys			
B. Has difficulty separating from parents, school, or babysitter			
C. Appears anxious or fearful of new people, situations			
D. Needs total control of the environment—"runs the show"			

continued

076-1643753-2

Infant/Toddler Symptom Checklist:
10 to 12 Months (continued)

How concerned are you about the symptoms you have checked above? (Circle one.)

Not concerned   Slightly concerned   Moderately concerned   Very concerned

---

Comments:

Infant/Toddler Symptom Checklist:
10 to 12 Months

Name________________________________ Date______________

	Never or Sometimes	Most Times	Past
1. Self-Regulation			
A. Is frequently irritable, fussy			
B. Goes easily from whimper to intense cry			
C. Is unable to wait for food or toy without crying or whining			
D. Demands adult company constantly			
E. Amount of time spent calming child during day (circle one): 15-30 minutes 1-2 hours 3 hours +			
2. Sleep			
A. Wakes 3 or more times in the night and is unable to fall back to sleep			
B. Requires extensive help to fall asleep; *specify:* rocking, long walks, stroking hair, car ride, other____________			
3. Eating or Feeding			
A. Gags or vomits			
4. Dressing, Bathing, Touch			
A. Resists cuddling, pulls away or arches			
B. Resists being placed in certain positions; for example, stomach or back			
C. Is distressed when clothes are removed			
5. Movement			
Is clumsy—falls, shows poor balance, bumps into things			
6. Listening, Language and Sound			
Is distracted by sounds not normally noticed by average person			
7. Looking and Sight			
Becomes excited in crowded, bustling settings such as supermarkets, restaurants			
8. Attachment/Emotional Functioning			
A. Avoids eye contact, turns away from the human face, prefers objects and toys			
B. Has difficulty separating from parents, school, or babysitter			
C. Appears anxious or fearful of new people, situations			
D. Needs total control of the environment—"runs the show"			

continued

076-1643753-2

Infant/Toddler Symptom Checklist:
10 to 12 Months (continued)

How concerned are you about the symptoms you have checked above? (Circle one.)

Not concerned   Slightly concerned   Moderately concerned   Very concerned

Comments:

Infant/Toddler Symptom Checklist:
10 to 12 Months

Name________________________ Date______________

	Never or Sometimes	Most Times	Past
1. Self-Regulation			
A. Is frequently irritable, fussy			
B. Goes easily from whimper to intense cry			
C. Is unable to wait for food or toy without crying or whining			
D. Demands adult company constantly			
E. Amount of time spent calming child during day (circle one): 15-30 minutes 1-2 hours 3 hours +			
2. Sleep			
A. Wakes 3 or more times in the night and is unable to fall back to sleep			
B. Requires extensive help to fall asleep; *specify:* rocking, long walks, stroking hair, car ride, other__________			
3. Eating or Feeding			
A. Gags or vomits			
4. Dressing, Bathing, Touch			
A. Resists cuddling, pulls away or arches			
B. Resists being placed in certain positions; for example, stomach or back			
C. Is distressed when clothes are removed			
5. Movement			
Is clumsy—falls, shows poor balance, bumps into things			
6. Listening, Language and Sound			
Is distracted by sounds not normally noticed by average person			
7. Looking and Sight			
Becomes excited in crowded, bustling settings such as supermarkets, restaurants			
8. Attachment/Emotional Functioning			
A. Avoids eye contact, turns away from the human face, prefers objects and toys			
B. Has difficulty separating from parents, school, or babysitter			
C. Appears anxious or fearful of new people, situations			
D. Needs total control of the environment—"runs the show"			

continued

076-1643753-2

Infant/Toddler Symptom Checklist:
10 to 12 Months (continued)

How concerned are you about the symptoms you have checked above? (Circle one.)

Not concerned   Slightly concerned   Moderately concerned   Very concerned

---

Comments:

Infant/Toddler Symptom Checklist: 10 to 12 Months

Name______________________________ Date______________

	Never or Sometimes	Most Times	Past
1. Self-Regulation			
A. Is frequently irritable, fussy			
B. Goes easily from whimper to intense cry			
C. Is unable to wait for food or toy without crying or whining			
D. Demands adult company constantly			
E. Amount of time spent calming child during day (circle one): 15-30 minutes 1-2 hours 3 hours +			
2. Sleep			
A. Wakes 3 or more times in the night and is unable to fall back to sleep			
B. Requires extensive help to fall asleep; *specify:* rocking, long walks, stroking hair, car ride, other__________			
3. Eating or Feeding			
A. Gags or vomits			
4. Dressing, Bathing, Touch			
A. Resists cuddling, pulls away or arches			
B. Resists being placed in certain positions; for example, stomach or back			
C. Is distressed when clothes are removed			
5. Movement			
Is clumsy—falls, shows poor balance, bumps into things			
6. Listening, Language and Sound			
Is distracted by sounds not normally noticed by average person			
7. Looking and Sight			
Becomes excited in crowded, bustling settings such as supermarkets, restaurants			
8. Attachment/Emotional Functioning			
A. Avoids eye contact, turns away from the human face, prefers objects and toys			
B. Has difficulty separating from parents, school, or babysitter			
C. Appears anxious or fearful of new people, situations			
D. Needs total control of the environment—"runs the show"			

continued

076-1643753-2

Infant/Toddler Symptom Checklist:
10 to 12 Months (continued)

How concerned are you about the symptoms you have checked above? (Circle one.)

Not concerned   Slightly concerned   Moderately concerned   Very concerned

---

Comments:

Infant/Toddler Symptom Checklist: 10 to 12 Months

Name________________________ Date______________

	Never or Sometimes	Most Times	Past
1. Self-Regulation			
A. Is frequently irritable, fussy			
B. Goes easily from whimper to intense cry			
C. Is unable to wait for food or toy without crying or whining			
D. Demands adult company constantly			
E. Amount of time spent calming child during day (circle one): 15-30 minutes 1-2 hours 3 hours +			
2. Sleep			
A. Wakes 3 or more times in the night and is unable to fall back to sleep			
B. Requires extensive help to fall asleep; *specify:* rocking, long walks, stroking hair, car ride, other__________			
3. Eating or Feeding			
A. Gags or vomits			
4. Dressing, Bathing, Touch			
A. Resists cuddling, pulls away or arches			
B. Resists being placed in certain positions; for example, stomach or back			
C. Is distressed when clothes are removed			
5. Movement			
Is clumsy—falls, shows poor balance, bumps into things			
6. Listening, Language and Sound			
Is distracted by sounds not normally noticed by average person			
7. Looking and Sight			
Becomes excited in crowded, bustling settings such as supermarkets, restaurants			
8. Attachment/Emotional Functioning			
A. Avoids eye contact, turns away from the human face, prefers objects and toys			
B. Has difficulty separating from parents, school, or babysitter			
C. Appears anxious or fearful of new people, situations			
D. Needs total control of the environment—"runs the show"			

continued

076-1643753-2

Infant/Toddler Symptom Checklist:
10 to 12 Months (continued)

How concerned are you about the symptoms you have checked above? (Circle one.)

Not concerned   Slightly concerned   Moderately concerned   Very concerned

---

Comments:

Infant/Toddler Symptom Checklist:
10 to 12 Months

Name______________________________ Date______________

	Never or Sometimes	Most Times	Past
1. Self-Regulation			
A. Is frequently irritable, fussy			
B. Goes easily from whimper to intense cry			
C. Is unable to wait for food or toy without crying or whining			
D. Demands adult company constantly			
E. Amount of time spent calming child during day (circle one): 15-30 minutes 1-2 hours 3 hours +			
2. Sleep			
A. Wakes 3 or more times in the night and is unable to fall back to sleep			
B. Requires extensive help to fall asleep; *specify:* rocking, long walks, stroking hair, car ride, other__________			
3. Eating or Feeding			
A. Gags or vomits			
4. Dressing, Bathing, Touch			
A. Resists cuddling, pulls away or arches			
B. Resists being placed in certain positions; for example, stomach or back			
C. Is distressed when clothes are removed			
5. Movement			
Is clumsy—falls, shows poor balance, bumps into things			
6. Listening, Language and Sound			
Is distracted by sounds not normally noticed by average person			
7. Looking and Sight			
Becomes excited in crowded, bustling settings such as supermarkets, restaurants			
8. Attachment/Emotional Functioning			
A. Avoids eye contact, turns away from the human face, prefers objects and toys			
B. Has difficulty separating from parents, school, or babysitter			
C. Appears anxious or fearful of new people, situations			
D. Needs total control of the environment—"runs the show"			

continued

076-1643753-2

How concerned are you about the symptoms you have checked above? (Circle one.)

Not concerned   Slightly concerned   Moderately concerned   Very concerned

Comments:

Infant/Toddler Symptom Checklist: 10 to 12 Months

Name________________________________ Date______________

	Never or Sometimes	Most Times	Past
1. Self-Regulation			
A. Is frequently irritable, fussy			
B. Goes easily from whimper to intense cry			
C. Is unable to wait for food or toy without crying or whining			
D. Demands adult company constantly			
E. Amount of time spent calming child during day (circle one): 15-30 minutes 1-2 hours 3 hours +			
2. Sleep			
A. Wakes 3 or more times in the night and is unable to fall back to sleep			
B. Requires extensive help to fall asleep; *specify:* rocking, long walks, stroking hair, car ride, other__________			
3. Eating or Feeding			
A. Gags or vomits			
4. Dressing, Bathing, Touch			
A. Resists cuddling, pulls away or arches			
B. Resists being placed in certain positions; for example, stomach or back			
C. Is distressed when clothes are removed			
5. Movement			
Is clumsy—falls, shows poor balance, bumps into things			
6. Listening, Language and Sound			
Is distracted by sounds not normally noticed by average person			
7. Looking and Sight			
Becomes excited in crowded, bustling settings such as supermarkets, restaurants			
8. Attachment/Emotional Functioning			
A. Avoids eye contact, turns away from the human face, prefers objects and toys			
B. Has difficulty separating from parents, school, or babysitter			
C. Appears anxious or fearful of new people, situations			
D. Needs total control of the environment—"runs the show"			

continued

076-1643753-2

Infant/Toddler Symptom Checklist:
10 to 12 Months (continued)

How concerned are you about the symptoms you have checked above? (Circle one.)

Not concerned   Slightly concerned   Moderately concerned   Very concerned

---

Comments:

Infant/Toddler Symptom Checklist:
10 to 12 Months

Name________________________ Date______________

	Never or Sometimes	Most Times	Past
1. Self-Regulation			
A. Is frequently irritable, fussy			
B. Goes easily from whimper to intense cry			
C. Is unable to wait for food or toy without crying or whining			
D. Demands adult company constantly			
E. Amount of time spent calming child during day (circle one): 15-30 minutes 1-2 hours 3 hours +			
2. Sleep			
A. Wakes 3 or more times in the night and is unable to fall back to sleep			
B. Requires extensive help to fall asleep; *specify:* rocking, long walks, stroking hair, car ride, other____________			
3. Eating or Feeding			
A. Gags or vomits			
4. Dressing, Bathing, Touch			
A. Resists cuddling, pulls away or arches			
B. Resists being placed in certain positions; for example, stomach or back			
C. Is distressed when clothes are removed			
5. Movement			
Is clumsy—falls, shows poor balance, bumps into things			
6. Listening, Language and Sound			
Is distracted by sounds not normally noticed by average person			
7. Looking and Sight			
Becomes excited in crowded, bustling settings such as supermarkets, restaurants			
8. Attachment/Emotional Functioning			
A. Avoids eye contact, turns away from the human face, prefers objects and toys			
B. Has difficulty separating from parents, school, or babysitter			
C. Appears anxious or fearful of new people, situations			
D. Needs total control of the environment—"runs the show"			

continued

076-1643753-2

Infant/Toddler Symptom Checklist:
10 to 12 Months (continued)

How concerned are you about the symptoms you have checked above? (Circle one.)

Not concerned   Slightly concerned   Moderately concerned   Very concerned

Comments:

Infant/Toddler Symptom Checklist: 10 to 12 Months

Name______________________________ Date______________

	Never or Sometimes	Most Times	Past
1. Self-Regulation			
A. Is frequently irritable, fussy			
B. Goes easily from whimper to intense cry			
C. Is unable to wait for food or toy without crying or whining			
D. Demands adult company constantly			
E. Amount of time spent calming child during day (circle one): 15-30 minutes 1-2 hours 3 hours +			
2. Sleep			
A. Wakes 3 or more times in the night and is unable to fall back to sleep			
B. Requires extensive help to fall asleep; *specify:* rocking, long walks, stroking hair, car ride, other____________			
3. Eating or Feeding			
A. Gags or vomits			
4. Dressing, Bathing, Touch			
A. Resists cuddling, pulls away or arches			
B. Resists being placed in certain positions; for example, stomach or back			
C. Is distressed when clothes are removed			
5. Movement			
Is clumsy—falls, shows poor balance, bumps into things			
6. Listening, Language and Sound			
Is distracted by sounds not normally noticed by average person			
7. Looking and Sight			
Becomes excited in crowded, bustling settings such as supermarkets, restaurants			
8. Attachment/Emotional Functioning			
A. Avoids eye contact, turns away from the human face, prefers objects and toys			
B. Has difficulty separating from parents, school, or babysitter			
C. Appears anxious or fearful of new people, situations			
D. Needs total control of the environment—"runs the show"			

continued

076-1643753-2

Infant/Toddler Symptom Checklist:
10 to 12 Months (continued)

How concerned are you about the symptoms you have checked above? (Circle one.)

Not concerned   Slightly concerned   Moderately concerned   Very concerned

---

Comments:

Infant/Toddler Symptom Checklist:
10 to 12 Months

Name________________________________ Date______________

	Never or Sometimes	Most Times	Past
1. Self-Regulation			
A. Is frequently irritable, fussy			
B. Goes easily from whimper to intense cry			
C. Is unable to wait for food or toy without crying or whining			
D. Demands adult company constantly			
E. Amount of time spent calming child during day (circle one): 15-30 minutes 1-2 hours 3 hours +			
2. Sleep			
A. Wakes 3 or more times in the night and is unable to fall back to sleep			
B. Requires extensive help to fall asleep; *specify:* rocking, long walks, stroking hair, car ride, other____________________			
3. Eating or Feeding			
A. Gags or vomits			
4. Dressing, Bathing, Touch			
A. Resists cuddling, pulls away or arches			
B. Resists being placed in certain positions; for example, stomach or back			
C. Is distressed when clothes are removed			
5. Movement			
Is clumsy—falls, shows poor balance, bumps into things			
6. Listening, Language and Sound			
Is distracted by sounds not normally noticed by average person			
7. Looking and Sight			
Becomes excited in crowded, bustling settings such as supermarkets, restaurants			
8. Attachment/Emotional Functioning			
A. Avoids eye contact, turns away from the human face, prefers objects and toys			
B. Has difficulty separating from parents, school, or babysitter			
C. Appears anxious or fearful of new people, situations			
D. Needs total control of the environment—"runs the show"			

continued

076-1643753-2

Infant/Toddler Symptom Checklist:
10 to 12 Months (continued)

How concerned are you about the symptoms you have checked above? (Circle one.)

Not concerned   Slightly concerned   Moderately concerned   Very concerned

Comments:

Infant/Toddler Symptom Checklist:
13 to 18 Months

Name________________________________ Date______________

	Never or Sometimes	Most Times	Past
1. Self-Regulation			
A. Is frequently irritable, fussy			
B. Goes easily from whimper to intense cry			
C. Can't calm self effectively by sucking on pacifier, looking at toys, or listening to caregiver			
D. Is unable to wait for food or toy without falling apart			
E. Can't change from one activity to another without distress			
F. Demands adult company constantly			
G. Amount of time spent calming child during day (circle one): 15-30 minutes 1-2 hours 3 hours +			
2. Attention			
A. Is easily distractible, shows fleeting attention			
B. Has difficulty paying attention, is difficult to reengage			
C. Is unable to shift focus easily from one object or activity to another			
3. Sleep			
A. Wakes 3 or more times in the night and is unable to fall back to sleep			
B. Requires extensive help to fall asleep; *specify:* rocking, long walks, stroking hair, car ride, other______________			
4. Dressing, Bathing, Touch			
A. Doesn't want to wear clothing			
B. Prefers certain clothing, complains that certain garments are too tight or scratchy			
C. Is distressed by having face or hair washed			
D. Resists cuddling, pulls away or arches			
E. Hates sitting in car seat			
F. Resists being placed in certain positions, such as stomach or back			
G. Is distressed when clothes removed			
5. Movement			
Craves swinging and moving upside-down			

continued

076-1643753-3

Infant/Toddler Symptom Checklist: 13 to18 Months (continued)

	Never or Sometimes	Most Times	Past
6. Listening, Language and Sound			
Startles or is distressed by loud sounds such as vacuum, doorbell, or barking dog			
7. Looking and Sight			
Becomes excited in crowded, bustling settings such as supermarkets, restaurants			
8. Attachment/Emotional Functioning			
A. Avoids eye contact, turns away from the human face, prefers objects and toys			
B. Does not appear happy			
C. Does not initiate interaction with caregiver: Parent needs to woo infant/child constantly			
D. Does not interact reciprocally (back-and-forth exchanges with caregiver)			
E. Has difficulty separating from parents, school, or babysitter			
F. Does not respond at all to limit setting, discipline			
G. Appears anxious or fearful of new people, situations			
H. Needs total control of the environment—"runs the show"			
I. Everyone has difficulty understanding the child's cues or emotions			

How concerned are you about the symptoms checked above? (Circle one.)

Not concerned Slightly concerned Moderately concerned Very concerned

Comments:

Infant/Toddler Symptom Checklist:
13 to 18 Months

Name______________________________ Date______________

	Never or Sometimes	Most Times	Past
1. Self-Regulation			
A. Is frequently irritable, fussy			
B. Goes easily from whimper to intense cry			
C. Can't calm self effectively by sucking on pacifier, looking at toys, or listening to caregiver			
D. Is unable to wait for food or toy without falling apart			
E. Can't change from one activity to another without distress			
F. Demands adult company constantly			
G. Amount of time spent calming child during day (circle one): 15-30 minutes 1-2 hours 3 hours +			
2. Attention			
A. Is easily distractible, shows fleeting attention			
B. Has difficulty paying attention, is difficult to reengage			
C. Is unable to shift focus easily from one object or activity to another			
3. Sleep			
A. Wakes 3 or more times in the night and is unable to fall back to sleep			
B. Requires extensive help to fall asleep; *specify:* rocking, long walks, stroking hair, car ride, other____________			
4. Dressing, Bathing, Touch			
A. Doesn't want to wear clothing			
B. Prefers certain clothing, complains that certain garments are too tight or scratchy			
C. Is distressed by having face or hair washed			
D. Resists cuddling, pulls away or arches			
E. Hates sitting in car seat			
F. Resists being placed in certain positions, such as stomach or back			
G. Is distressed when clothes removed			
5. Movement			
Craves swinging and moving upside-down			

continued

076-1643753-3

Infant/Toddler Symptom Checklist: 13 to18 Months (continued)

	Never or Sometimes	Most Times	Past
6. Listening, Language and Sound			
Startles or is distressed by loud sounds such as vacuum, doorbell, or barking dog			
7. Looking and Sight			
Becomes excited in crowded, bustling settings such as supermarkets, restaurants			
8. Attachment/Emotional Functioning			
A. Avoids eye contact, turns away from the human face, prefers objects and toys			
B. Does not appear happy			
C. Does not initiate interaction with caregiver: Parent needs to woo infant/child constantly			
D. Does not interact reciprocally (back-and-forth exchanges with caregiver)			
E. Has difficulty separating from parents, school, or babysitter			
F. Does not respond at all to limit setting, discipline			
G. Appears anxious or fearful of new people, situations			
H. Needs total control of the environment—"runs the show"			
I. Everyone has difficulty understanding the child's cues or emotions			

How concerned are you about the symptoms checked above? (Circle one.)

Not concerned Slightly concerned Moderately concerned Very concerned

Comments:

Infant/Toddler Symptom Checklist: 13 to 18 Months

Name______________________________ Date____________

	Never or Sometimes	Most Times	Past
1. Self-Regulation			
A. Is frequently irritable, fussy			
B. Goes easily from whimper to intense cry			
C. Can't calm self effectively by sucking on pacifier, looking at toys, or listening to caregiver			
D. Is unable to wait for food or toy without falling apart			
E. Can't change from one activity to another without distress			
F. Demands adult company constantly			
G. Amount of time spent calming child during day (circle one): 15-30 minutes 1-2 hours 3 hours +			
2. Attention			
A. Is easily distractible, shows fleeting attention			
B. Has difficulty paying attention, is difficult to reengage			
C. Is unable to shift focus easily from one object or activity to another			
3. Sleep			
A. Wakes 3 or more times in the night and is unable to fall back to sleep			
B. Requires extensive help to fall asleep; *specify:* rocking, long walks, stroking hair, car ride, other____________			
4. Dressing, Bathing, Touch			
A. Doesn't want to wear clothing			
B. Prefers certain clothing, complains that certain garments are too tight or scratchy			
C. Is distressed by having face or hair washed			
D. Resists cuddling, pulls away or arches			
E. Hates sitting in car seat			
F. Resists being placed in certain positions, such as stomach or back			
G. Is distressed when clothes removed			
5. Movement			
Craves swinging and moving upside-down			

continued

076-1643753-3

Infant/Toddler Symptom Checklist:
13 to18 Months (continued)

	Never or Sometimes	Most Times	Past
6. Listening, Language and Sound			
Startles or is distressed by loud sounds such as vacuum, doorbell, or barking dog			
7. Looking and Sight			
Becomes excited in crowded, bustling settings such as supermarkets, restaurants			
8. Attachment/Emotional Functioning			
A. Avoids eye contact, turns away from the human face, prefers objects and toys			
B. Does not appear happy			
C. Does not initiate interaction with caregiver: Parent needs to woo infant/child constantly			
D. Does not interact reciprocally (back-and-forth exchanges with caregiver)			
E. Has difficulty separating from parents, school, or babysitter			
F. Does not respond at all to limit setting, discipline			
G. Appears anxious or fearful of new people, situations			
H. Needs total control of the environment—"runs the show"			
I. Everyone has difficulty understanding the child's cues or emotions			

How concerned are you about the symptoms checked above? (Circle one.)

Not concerned   Slightly concerned   Moderately concerned   Very concerned

Comments:

Infant/Toddler Symptom Checklist:
13 to 18 Months

Name________________________________ Date______________

	Never or Sometimes	Most Times	Past
1. Self-Regulation			
A. Is frequently irritable, fussy			
B. Goes easily from whimper to intense cry			
C. Can't calm self effectively by sucking on pacifier, looking at toys, or listening to caregiver			
D. Is unable to wait for food or toy without falling apart			
E. Can't change from one activity to another without distress			
F. Demands adult company constantly			
G. Amount of time spent calming child during day (circle one): 15-30 minutes 1-2 hours 3 hours +			
2. Attention			
A. Is easily distractible, shows fleeting attention			
B. Has difficulty paying attention, is difficult to reengage			
C. Is unable to shift focus easily from one object or activity to another			
3. Sleep			
A. Wakes 3 or more times in the night and is unable to fall back to sleep			
B. Requires extensive help to fall asleep; *specify:* rocking, long walks, stroking hair, car ride, other__________			
4. Dressing, Bathing, Touch			
A. Doesn't want to wear clothing			
B. Prefers certain clothing, complains that certain garments are too tight or scratchy			
C. Is distressed by having face or hair washed			
D. Resists cuddling, pulls away or arches			
E. Hates sitting in car seat			
F. Resists being placed in certain positions, such as stomach or back			
G. Is distressed when clothes removed			
5. Movement			
Craves swinging and moving upside-down			

continued

076-1643753-3

Infant/Toddler Symptom Checklist: 13 to18 Months (continued)

	Never or Sometimes	Most Times	Past
6. Listening, Language and Sound			
Startles or is distressed by loud sounds such as vacuum, doorbell, or barking dog			
7. Looking and Sight			
Becomes excited in crowded, bustling settings such as supermarkets, restaurants			
8. Attachment/Emotional Functioning			
A. Avoids eye contact, turns away from the human face, prefers objects and toys			
B. Does not appear happy			
C. Does not initiate interaction with caregiver: Parent needs to woo infant/child constantly			
D. Does not interact reciprocally (back-and-forth exchanges with caregiver)			
E. Has difficulty separating from parents, school, or babysitter			
F. Does not respond at all to limit setting, discipline			
G. Appears anxious or fearful of new people, situations			
H. Needs total control of the environment—"runs the show"			
I. Everyone has difficulty understanding the child's cues or emotions			

How concerned are you about the symptoms checked above? (Circle one.)

Not concerned   Slightly concerned   Moderately concerned   Very concerned

Comments:

Infant/Toddler Symptom Checklist:
13 to 18 Months

Name______________________________ Date______________

	Never or Sometimes	Most Times	Past
1. Self-Regulation			
A. Is frequently irritable, fussy			
B. Goes easily from whimper to intense cry			
C. Can't calm self effectively by sucking on pacifier, looking at toys, or listening to caregiver			
D. Is unable to wait for food or toy without falling apart			
E. Can't change from one activity to another without distress			
F. Demands adult company constantly			
G. Amount of time spent calming child during day (circle one): 15-30 minutes 1-2 hours 3 hours +			
2. Attention			
A. Is easily distractible, shows fleeting attention			
B. Has difficulty paying attention, is difficult to reengage			
C. Is unable to shift focus easily from one object or activity to another			
3. Sleep			
A. Wakes 3 or more times in the night and is unable to fall back to sleep			
B. Requires extensive help to fall asleep; *specify:* rocking, long walks, stroking hair, car ride, other__________			
4. Dressing, Bathing, Touch			
A. Doesn't want to wear clothing			
B. Prefers certain clothing, complains that certain garments are too tight or scratchy			
C. Is distressed by having face or hair washed			
D. Resists cuddling, pulls away or arches			
E. Hates sitting in car seat			
F. Resists being placed in certain positions, such as stomach or back			
G. Is distressed when clothes removed			
5. Movement			
Craves swinging and moving upside-down			

continued

076-1643753-3

Infant/Toddler Symptom Checklist:
13 to18 Months (continued)

	Never or Sometimes	Most Times	Past
6. Listening, Language and Sound			
Startles or is distressed by loud sounds such as vacuum, doorbell, or barking dog			
7. Looking and Sight			
Becomes excited in crowded, bustling settings such as supermarkets, restaurants			
8. Attachment/Emotional Functioning			
A. Avoids eye contact, turns away from the human face, prefers objects and toys			
B. Does not appear happy			
C. Does not initiate interaction with caregiver: Parent needs to woo infant/child constantly			
D. Does not interact reciprocally (back-and-forth exchanges with caregiver)			
E. Has difficulty separating from parents, school, or babysitter			
F. Does not respond at all to limit setting, discipline			
G. Appears anxious or fearful of new people, situations			
H. Needs total control of the environment—"runs the show"			
I. Everyone has difficulty understanding the child's cues or emotions			

How concerned are you about the symptoms checked above? (Circle one.)

Not concerned   Slightly concerned   Moderately concerned   Very concerned

Comments:

Infant/Toddler Symptom Checklist:
13 to 18 Months

Name____________________ Date__________

	Never or Sometimes	Most Times	Past
1. Self-Regulation			
A. Is frequently irritable, fussy			
B. Goes easily from whimper to intense cry			
C. Can't calm self effectively by sucking on pacifier, looking at toys, or listening to caregiver			
D. Is unable to wait for food or toy without falling apart			
E. Can't change from one activity to another without distress			
F. Demands adult company constantly			
G. Amount of time spent calming child during day (circle one): 15-30 minutes 1-2 hours 3 hours +			
2. Attention			
A. Is easily distractible, shows fleeting attention			
B. Has difficulty paying attention, is difficult to reengage			
C. Is unable to shift focus easily from one object or activity to another			
3. Sleep			
A. Wakes 3 or more times in the night and is unable to fall back to sleep			
B. Requires extensive help to fall asleep; *specify:* rocking, long walks, stroking hair, car ride, other__________			
4. Dressing, Bathing, Touch			
A. Doesn't want to wear clothing			
B. Prefers certain clothing, complains that certain garments are too tight or scratchy			
C. Is distressed by having face or hair washed			
D. Resists cuddling, pulls away or arches			
E. Hates sitting in car seat			
F. Resists being placed in certain positions, such as stomach or back			
G. Is distressed when clothes removed			
5. Movement			
Craves swinging and moving upside-down			

continued

076-1643753-3

Infant/Toddler Symptom Checklist: 13 to18 Months (continued)

	Never or Sometimes	Most Times	Past
6. Listening, Language and Sound			
Startles or is distressed by loud sounds such as vacuum, doorbell, or barking dog			
7. Looking and Sight			
Becomes excited in crowded, bustling settings such as supermarkets, restaurants			
8. Attachment/Emotional Functioning			
A. Avoids eye contact, turns away from the human face, prefers objects and toys			
B. Does not appear happy			
C. Does not initiate interaction with caregiver: Parent needs to woo infant/child constantly			
D. Does not interact reciprocally (back-and-forth exchanges with caregiver)			
E. Has difficulty separating from parents, school, or babysitter			
F. Does not respond at all to limit setting, discipline			
G. Appears anxious or fearful of new people, situations			
H. Needs total control of the environment—"runs the show"			
I. Everyone has difficulty understanding the child's cues or emotions			

How concerned are you about the symptoms checked above? (Circle one.)

Not concerned Slightly concerned Moderately concerned Very concerned

Comments:

Infant/Toddler Symptom Checklist: 13 to 18 Months

Name______________________ Date__________

	Never or Sometimes	Most Times	Past
1. Self-Regulation			
A. Is frequently irritable, fussy			
B. Goes easily from whimper to intense cry			
C. Can't calm self effectively by sucking on pacifier, looking at toys, or listening to caregiver			
D. Is unable to wait for food or toy without falling apart			
E. Can't change from one activity to another without distress			
F. Demands adult company constantly			
G. Amount of time spent calming child during day (circle one): 15-30 minutes 1-2 hours 3 hours +			
2. Attention			
A. Is easily distractible, shows fleeting attention			
B. Has difficulty paying attention, is difficult to reengage			
C. Is unable to shift focus easily from one object or activity to another			
3. Sleep			
A. Wakes 3 or more times in the night and is unable to fall back to sleep			
B. Requires extensive help to fall asleep; *specify:* rocking, long walks, stroking hair, car ride, other__________			
4. Dressing, Bathing, Touch			
A. Doesn't want to wear clothing			
B. Prefers certain clothing, complains that certain garments are too tight or scratchy			
C. Is distressed by having face or hair washed			
D. Resists cuddling, pulls away or arches			
E. Hates sitting in car seat			
F. Resists being placed in certain positions, such as stomach or back			
G. Is distressed when clothes removed			
5. Movement			
Craves swinging and moving upside-down			

continued

Infant/Toddler Symptom Checklist: 13 to18 Months (continued)

	Never or Sometimes	Most Times	Past
6. Listening, Language and Sound			
Startles or is distressed by loud sounds such as vacuum, doorbell, or barking dog			
7. Looking and Sight			
Becomes excited in crowded, bustling settings such as supermarkets, restaurants			
8. Attachment/Emotional Functioning			
A. Avoids eye contact, turns away from the human face, prefers objects and toys			
B. Does not appear happy			
C. Does not initiate interaction with caregiver: Parent needs to woo infant/child constantly			
D. Does not interact reciprocally (back-and-forth exchanges with caregiver)			
E. Has difficulty separating from parents, school, or babysitter			
F. Does not respond at all to limit setting, discipline			
G. Appears anxious or fearful of new people, situations			
H. Needs total control of the environment—"runs the show"			
I. Everyone has difficulty understanding the child's cues or emotions			

How concerned are you about the symptoms checked above? (Circle one.)

Not concerned   Slightly concerned   Moderately concerned   Very concerned

Comments:

Infant/Toddler Symptom Checklist:
13 to 18 Months

Name_______________________________________ Date______________

	Never or Sometimes	Most Times	Past
1. Self-Regulation			
A. Is frequently irritable, fussy			
B. Goes easily from whimper to intense cry			
C. Can't calm self effectively by sucking on pacifier, looking at toys, or listening to caregiver			
D. Is unable to wait for food or toy without falling apart			
E. Can't change from one activity to another without distress			
F. Demands adult company constantly			
G. Amount of time spent calming child during day (circle one): 15-30 minutes 1-2 hours 3 hours +			
2. Attention			
A. Is easily distractible, shows fleeting attention			
B. Has difficulty paying attention, is difficult to reengage			
C. Is unable to shift focus easily from one object or activity to another			
3. Sleep			
A. Wakes 3 or more times in the night and is unable to fall back to sleep			
B. Requires extensive help to fall asleep; *specify:* rocking, long walks, stroking hair, car ride, other_______________			
4. Dressing, Bathing, Touch			
A. Doesn't want to wear clothing			
B. Prefers certain clothing, complains that certain garments are too tight or scratchy			
C. Is distressed by having face or hair washed			
D. Resists cuddling, pulls away or arches			
E. Hates sitting in car seat			
F. Resists being placed in certain positions, such as stomach or back			
G. Is distressed when clothes removed			
5. Movement			
Craves swinging and moving upside-down			

continued

076-1643753-3

Infant/Toddler Symptom Checklist:
13 to18 Months (continued)

	Never or Sometimes	Most Times	Past
6. Listening, Language and Sound			
Startles or is distressed by loud sounds such as vacuum, doorbell, or barking dog			
7. Looking and Sight			
Becomes excited in crowded, bustling settings such as supermarkets, restaurants			
8. Attachment/Emotional Functioning			
A. Avoids eye contact, turns away from the human face, prefers objects and toys			
B. Does not appear happy			
C. Does not initiate interaction with caregiver: Parent needs to woo infant/child constantly			
D. Does not interact reciprocally (back-and-forth exchanges with caregiver)			
E. Has difficulty separating from parents, school, or babysitter			
F. Does not respond at all to limit setting, discipline			
G. Appears anxious or fearful of new people, situations			
H. Needs total control of the environment—"runs the show"			
I. Everyone has difficulty understanding the child's cues or emotions			

How concerned are you about the symptoms checked above? (Circle one.)

Not concerned   Slightly concerned   Moderately concerned   Very concerned

Comments:

Infant/Toddler Symptom Checklist:
13 to 18 Months

Name______________________________ Date______________

	Never or Sometimes	Most Times	Past
1. Self-Regulation			
A. Is frequently irritable, fussy			
B. Goes easily from whimper to intense cry			
C. Can't calm self effectively by sucking on pacifier, looking at toys, or listening to caregiver			
D. Is unable to wait for food or toy without falling apart			
E. Can't change from one activity to another without distress			
F. Demands adult company constantly			
G. Amount of time spent calming child during day (circle one): 15-30 minutes 1-2 hours 3 hours +			
2. Attention			
A. Is easily distractible, shows fleeting attention			
B. Has difficulty paying attention, is difficult to reengage			
C. Is unable to shift focus easily from one object or activity to another			
3. Sleep			
A. Wakes 3 or more times in the night and is unable to fall back to sleep			
B. Requires extensive help to fall asleep; *specify:* rocking, long walks, stroking hair, car ride, other__________			
4. Dressing, Bathing, Touch			
A. Doesn't want to wear clothing			
B. Prefers certain clothing, complains that certain garments are too tight or scratchy			
C. Is distressed by having face or hair washed			
D. Resists cuddling, pulls away or arches			
E. Hates sitting in car seat			
F. Resists being placed in certain positions, such as stomach or back			
G. Is distressed when clothes removed			
5. Movement			
Craves swinging and moving upside-down			

continued

076-1643753-3

Infant/Toddler Symptom Checklist: 13 to18 Months (continued)

	Never or Sometimes	Most Times	Past
6. Listening, Language and Sound			
Startles or is distressed by loud sounds such as vacuum, doorbell, or barking dog			
7. Looking and Sight			
Becomes excited in crowded, bustling settings such as supermarkets, restaurants			
8. Attachment/Emotional Functioning			
A. Avoids eye contact, turns away from the human face, prefers objects and toys			
B. Does not appear happy			
C. Does not initiate interaction with caregiver: Parent needs to woo infant/child constantly			
D. Does not interact reciprocally (back-and-forth exchanges with caregiver)			
E. Has difficulty separating from parents, school, or babysitter			
F. Does not respond at all to limit setting, discipline			
G. Appears anxious or fearful of new people, situations			
H. Needs total control of the environment—"runs the show"			
I. Everyone has difficulty understanding the child's cues or emotions			

How concerned are you about the symptoms checked above? (Circle one.)

Not concerned   Slightly concerned   Moderately concerned   Very concerned

Comments:

Infant/Toddler Symptom Checklist:
13 to 18 Months

Name________________________ Date____________

	Never or Sometimes	Most Times	Past
1. Self-Regulation			
A. Is frequently irritable, fussy			
B. Goes easily from whimper to intense cry			
C. Can't calm self effectively by sucking on pacifier, looking at toys, or listening to caregiver			
D. Is unable to wait for food or toy without falling apart			
E. Can't change from one activity to another without distress			
F. Demands adult company constantly			
G. Amount of time spent calming child during day (circle one): 15-30 minutes 1-2 hours 3 hours +			
2. Attention			
A. Is easily distractible, shows fleeting attention			
B. Has difficulty paying attention, is difficult to reengage			
C. Is unable to shift focus easily from one object or activity to another			
3. Sleep			
A. Wakes 3 or more times in the night and is unable to fall back to sleep			
B. Requires extensive help to fall asleep; *specify:* rocking, long walks, stroking hair, car ride, other__________			
4. Dressing, Bathing, Touch			
A. Doesn't want to wear clothing			
B. Prefers certain clothing, complains that certain garments are too tight or scratchy			
C. Is distressed by having face or hair washed			
D. Resists cuddling, pulls away or arches			
E. Hates sitting in car seat			
F. Resists being placed in certain positions, such as stomach or back			
G. Is distressed when clothes removed			
5. Movement			
Craves swinging and moving upside-down			

continued

076-1643753-3

Infant/Toddler Symptom Checklist:
13 to18 Months (continued)

	Never or Sometimes	Most Times	Past
6. Listening, Language and Sound			
Startles or is distressed by loud sounds such as vacuum, doorbell, or barking dog			
7. Looking and Sight			
Becomes excited in crowded, bustling settings such as supermarkets, restaurants			
8. Attachment/Emotional Functioning			
A. Avoids eye contact, turns away from the human face, prefers objects and toys			
B. Does not appear happy			
C. Does not initiate interaction with caregiver: Parent needs to woo infant/child constantly			
D. Does not interact reciprocally (back-and-forth exchanges with caregiver)			
E. Has difficulty separating from parents, school, or babysitter			
F. Does not respond at all to limit setting, discipline			
G. Appears anxious or fearful of new people, situations			
H. Needs total control of the environment—"runs the show"			
I. Everyone has difficulty understanding the child's cues or emotions			

How concerned are you about the symptoms checked above? (Circle one.)

Not concerned   Slightly concerned   Moderately concerned   Very concerned

Comments:

Infant/Toddler Symptom Checklist:
13 to 18 Months

Name______________________________ Date______________

	Never or Sometimes	Most Times	Past
1. Self-Regulation			
A. Is frequently irritable, fussy			
B. Goes easily from whimper to intense cry			
C. Can't calm self effectively by sucking on pacifier, looking at toys, or listening to caregiver			
D. Is unable to wait for food or toy without falling apart			
E. Can't change from one activity to another without distress			
F. Demands adult company constantly			
G. Amount of time spent calming child during day (circle one): 15-30 minutes 1-2 hours 3 hours +			
2. Attention			
A. Is easily distractible, shows fleeting attention			
B. Has difficulty paying attention, is difficult to reengage			
C. Is unable to shift focus easily from one object or activity to another			
3. Sleep			
A. Wakes 3 or more times in the night and is unable to fall back to sleep			
B. Requires extensive help to fall asleep; *specify:* rocking, long walks, stroking hair, car ride, other__________________			
4. Dressing, Bathing, Touch			
A. Doesn't want to wear clothing			
B. Prefers certain clothing, complains that certain garments are too tight or scratchy			
C. Is distressed by having face or hair washed			
D. Resists cuddling, pulls away or arches			
E. Hates sitting in car seat			
F. Resists being placed in certain positions, such as stomach or back			
G. Is distressed when clothes removed			
5. Movement			
Craves swinging and moving upside-down			

continued

076-1643753-3

Infant/Toddler Symptom Checklist: 13 to18 Months (continued)

	Never or Sometimes	Most Times	Past
6. Listening, Language and Sound			
Startles or is distressed by loud sounds such as vacuum, doorbell, or barking dog			
7. Looking and Sight			
Becomes excited in crowded, bustling settings such as supermarkets, restaurants			
8. Attachment/Emotional Functioning			
A. Avoids eye contact, turns away from the human face, prefers objects and toys			
B. Does not appear happy			
C. Does not initiate interaction with caregiver: Parent needs to woo infant/child constantly			
D. Does not interact reciprocally (back-and-forth exchanges with caregiver)			
E. Has difficulty separating from parents, school, or babysitter			
F. Does not respond at all to limit setting, discipline			
G. Appears anxious or fearful of new people, situations			
H. Needs total control of the environment—"runs the show"			
I. Everyone has difficulty understanding the child's cues or emotions			

How concerned are you about the symptoms checked above? (Circle one.)

Not concerned   Slightly concerned   Moderately concerned   Very concerned

Comments:

Infant/Toddler Symptom Checklist: 13 to 18 Months

Name____ Date_______________

	Never or Sometimes	Most Times	Past
1. Self-Regulation			
A. Is frequently irritable, fussy			
B. Goes easily from whimper to intense cry			
C. Can't calm self effectively by sucking on pacifier, looking at toys, or listening to caregiver			
D. Is unable to wait for food or toy without falling apart			
E. Can't change from one activity to another without distress			
F. Demands adult company constantly			
G. Amount of time spent calming child during day (circle one): 15-30 minutes 1-2 hours 3 hours +			
2. Attention			
A. Is easily distractible, shows fleeting attention			
B. Has difficulty paying attention, is difficult to reengage			
C. Is unable to shift focus easily from one object or activity to another			
3. Sleep			
A. Wakes 3 or more times in the night and is unable to fall back to sleep			
B. Requires extensive help to fall asleep; *specify:* rocking, long walks, stroking hair, car ride, other___________________			
4. Dressing, Bathing, Touch			
A. Doesn't want to wear clothing			
B. Prefers certain clothing, complains that certain garments are too tight or scratchy			
C. Is distressed by having face or hair washed			
D. Resists cuddling, pulls away or arches			
E. Hates sitting in car seat			
F. Resists being placed in certain positions, such as stomach or back			
G. Is distressed when clothes removed			
5. Movement			
Craves swinging and moving upside-down			

continued

076-1643753-3

Infant/Toddler Symptom Checklist:
13 to18 Months (continued)

	Never or Sometimes	Most Times	Past
6. Listening, Language and Sound			
Startles or is distressed by loud sounds such as vacuum, doorbell, or barking dog			
7. Looking and Sight			
Becomes excited in crowded, bustling settings such as supermarkets, restaurants			
8. Attachment/Emotional Functioning			
A. Avoids eye contact, turns away from the human face, prefers objects and toys			
B. Does not appear happy			
C. Does not initiate interaction with caregiver: Parent needs to woo infant/child constantly			
D. Does not interact reciprocally (back-and-forth exchanges with caregiver)			
E. Has difficulty separating from parents, school, or babysitter			
F. Does not respond at all to limit setting, discipline			
G. Appears anxious or fearful of new people, situations			
H. Needs total control of the environment—"runs the show"			
I. Everyone has difficulty understanding the child's cues or emotions			

How concerned are you about the symptoms checked above? (Circle one.)

Not concerned   Slightly concerned   Moderately concerned   Very concerned

Comments:

Infant/Toddler Symptom Checklist: 13 to 18 Months

Name__________________________ Date______________

	Never or Sometimes	Most Times	Past
1. Self-Regulation			
A. Is frequently irritable, fussy			
B. Goes easily from whimper to intense cry			
C. Can't calm self effectively by sucking on pacifier, looking at toys, or listening to caregiver			
D. Is unable to wait for food or toy without falling apart			
E. Can't change from one activity to another without distress			
F. Demands adult company constantly			
G. Amount of time spent calming child during day (circle one): 15-30 minutes 1-2 hours 3 hours +			
2. Attention			
A. Is easily distractible, shows fleeting attention			
B. Has difficulty paying attention, is difficult to reengage			
C. Is unable to shift focus easily from one object or activity to another			
3. Sleep			
A. Wakes 3 or more times in the night and is unable to fall back to sleep			
B. Requires extensive help to fall asleep; *specify:* rocking, long walks, stroking hair, car ride, other__________			
4. Dressing, Bathing, Touch			
A. Doesn't want to wear clothing			
B. Prefers certain clothing, complains that certain garments are too tight or scratchy			
C. Is distressed by having face or hair washed			
D. Resists cuddling, pulls away or arches			
E. Hates sitting in car seat			
F. Resists being placed in certain positions, such as stomach or back			
G. Is distressed when clothes removed			
5. Movement			
Craves swinging and moving upside-down			

continued

076-1643753-3

Infant/Toddler Symptom Checklist: 13 to18 Months (continued)

	Never or Sometimes	Most Times	Past
6. Listening, Language and Sound			
Startles or is distressed by loud sounds such as vacuum, doorbell, or barking dog			
7. Looking and Sight			
Becomes excited in crowded, bustling settings such as supermarkets, restaurants			
8. Attachment/Emotional Functioning			
A. Avoids eye contact, turns away from the human face, prefers objects and toys			
B. Does not appear happy			
C. Does not initiate interaction with caregiver: Parent needs to woo infant/child constantly			
D. Does not interact reciprocally (back-and-forth exchanges with caregiver)			
E. Has difficulty separating from parents, school, or babysitter			
F. Does not respond at all to limit setting, discipline			
G. Appears anxious or fearful of new people, situations			
H. Needs total control of the environment—"runs the show"			
I. Everyone has difficulty understanding the child's cues or emotions			

How concerned are you about the symptoms checked above? (Circle one.)

Not concerned   Slightly concerned   Moderately concerned   Very concerned

Comments:

Infant/Toddler Symptom Checklist:
13 to 18 Months

Name______________________________ Date______________

	Never or Sometimes	Most Times	Past
1. Self-Regulation			
A. Is frequently irritable, fussy			
B. Goes easily from whimper to intense cry			
C. Can't calm self effectively by sucking on pacifier, looking at toys, or listening to caregiver			
D. Is unable to wait for food or toy without falling apart			
E. Can't change from one activity to another without distress			
F. Demands adult company constantly			
G. Amount of time spent calming child during day (circle one): 15-30 minutes 1-2 hours 3 hours +			
2. Attention			
A. Is easily distractible, shows fleeting attention			
B. Has difficulty paying attention, is difficult to reengage			
C. Is unable to shift focus easily from one object or activity to another			
3. Sleep			
A. Wakes 3 or more times in the night and is unable to fall back to sleep			
B. Requires extensive help to fall asleep; *specify:* rocking, long walks, stroking hair, car ride, other____________			
4. Dressing, Bathing, Touch			
A. Doesn't want to wear clothing			
B. Prefers certain clothing, complains that certain garments are too tight or scratchy			
C. Is distressed by having face or hair washed			
D. Resists cuddling, pulls away or arches			
E. Hates sitting in car seat			
F. Resists being placed in certain positions, such as stomach or back			
G. Is distressed when clothes removed			
5. Movement			
Craves swinging and moving upside-down			

continued

076-1643753-3

Infant/Toddler Symptom Checklist: 13 to18 Months (continued)

	Never or Sometimes	Most Times	Past
6. Listening, Language and Sound			
Startles or is distressed by loud sounds such as vacuum, doorbell, or barking dog			
7. Looking and Sight			
Becomes excited in crowded, bustling settings such as supermarkets, restaurants			
8. Attachment/Emotional Functioning			
A. Avoids eye contact, turns away from the human face, prefers objects and toys			
B. Does not appear happy			
C. Does not initiate interaction with caregiver: Parent needs to woo infant/child constantly			
D. Does not interact reciprocally (back-and-forth exchanges with caregiver)			
E. Has difficulty separating from parents, school, or babysitter			
F. Does not respond at all to limit setting, discipline			
G. Appears anxious or fearful of new people, situations			
H. Needs total control of the environment—"runs the show"			
I. Everyone has difficulty understanding the child's cues or emotions			

How concerned are you about the symptoms checked above? (Circle one.)

Not concerned Slightly concerned Moderately concerned Very concerned

Comments:

Infant/Toddler Symptom Checklist:
13 to 18 Months

Name____________________________ Date______________

	Never or Sometimes	Most Times	Past
1. Self-Regulation			
A. Is frequently irritable, fussy			
B. Goes easily from whimper to intense cry			
C. Can't calm self effectively by sucking on pacifier, looking at toys, or listening to caregiver			
D. Is unable to wait for food or toy without falling apart			
E. Can't change from one activity to another without distress			
F. Demands adult company constantly			
G. Amount of time spent calming child during day (circle one): 15-30 minutes 1-2 hours 3 hours +			
2. Attention			
A. Is easily distractible, shows fleeting attention			
B. Has difficulty paying attention, is difficult to reengage			
C. Is unable to shift focus easily from one object or activity to another			
3. Sleep			
A. Wakes 3 or more times in the night and is unable to fall back to sleep			
B. Requires extensive help to fall asleep; *specify:* rocking, long walks, stroking hair, car ride, other__________			
4. Dressing, Bathing, Touch			
A. Doesn't want to wear clothing			
B. Prefers certain clothing, complains that certain garments are too tight or scratchy			
C. Is distressed by having face or hair washed			
D. Resists cuddling, pulls away or arches			
E. Hates sitting in car seat			
F. Resists being placed in certain positions, such as stomach or back			
G. Is distressed when clothes removed			
5. Movement			
Craves swinging and moving upside-down			

continued

076-1643753-3

Infant/Toddler Symptom Checklist: 13 to18 Months (continued)

	Never or Sometimes	Most Times	Past
6. Listening, Language and Sound			
Startles or is distressed by loud sounds such as vacuum, doorbell, or barking dog			
7. Looking and Sight			
Becomes excited in crowded, bustling settings such as supermarkets, restaurants			
8. Attachment/Emotional Functioning			
A. Avoids eye contact, turns away from the human face, prefers objects and toys			
B. Does not appear happy			
C. Does not initiate interaction with caregiver: Parent needs to woo infant/child constantly			
D. Does not interact reciprocally (back-and-forth exchanges with caregiver)			
E. Has difficulty separating from parents, school, or babysitter			
F. Does not respond at all to limit setting, discipline			
G. Appears anxious or fearful of new people, situations			
H. Needs total control of the environment—"runs the show"			
I. Everyone has difficulty understanding the child's cues or emotions			

How concerned are you about the symptoms checked above? (Circle one.)

Not concerned   Slightly concerned   Moderately concerned   Very concerned

Comments:

Infant/Toddler Symptom Checklist:
13 to 18 Months

Name______________________________ Date______________

	Never or Sometimes	Most Times	Past
1. Self-Regulation			
A. Is frequently irritable, fussy			
B. Goes easily from whimper to intense cry			
C. Can't calm self effectively by sucking on pacifier, looking at toys, or listening to caregiver			
D. Is unable to wait for food or toy without falling apart			
E. Can't change from one activity to another without distress			
F. Demands adult company constantly			
G. Amount of time spent calming child during day (circle one): 15-30 minutes 1-2 hours 3 hours +			
2. Attention			
A. Is easily distractible, shows fleeting attention			
B. Has difficulty paying attention, is difficult to reengage			
C. Is unable to shift focus easily from one object or activity to another			
3. Sleep			
A. Wakes 3 or more times in the night and is unable to fall back to sleep			
B. Requires extensive help to fall asleep; *specify:* rocking, long walks, stroking hair, car ride, other___________			
4. Dressing, Bathing, Touch			
A. Doesn't want to wear clothing			
B. Prefers certain clothing, complains that certain garments are too tight or scratchy			
C. Is distressed by having face or hair washed			
D. Resists cuddling, pulls away or arches			
E. Hates sitting in car seat			
F. Resists being placed in certain positions, such as stomach or back			
G. Is distressed when clothes removed			
5. Movement			
Craves swinging and moving upside-down			

continued

076-1643753-3

Infant/Toddler Symptom Checklist:
13 to18 Months (continued)

	Never or Sometimes	Most Times	Past
6. Listening, Language and Sound			
Startles or is distressed by loud sounds such as vacuum, doorbell, or barking dog			
7. Looking and Sight			
Becomes excited in crowded, bustling settings such as supermarkets, restaurants			
8. Attachment/Emotional Functioning			
A. Avoids eye contact, turns away from the human face, prefers objects and toys			
B. Does not appear happy			
C. Does not initiate interaction with caregiver: Parent needs to woo infant/child constantly			
D. Does not interact reciprocally (back-and-forth exchanges with caregiver)			
E. Has difficulty separating from parents, school, or babysitter			
F. Does not respond at all to limit setting, discipline			
G. Appears anxious or fearful of new people, situations			
H. Needs total control of the environment—"runs the show"			
I. Everyone has difficulty understanding the child's cues or emotions			

How concerned are you about the symptoms checked above? (Circle one.)

Not concerned   Slightly concerned   Moderately concerned   Very concerned

Comments:

Infant/Toddler Symptom Checklist:
13 to 18 Months

Name________________________ Date____________

	Never or Sometimes	Most Times	Past
1. Self-Regulation			
A. Is frequently irritable, fussy			
B. Goes easily from whimper to intense cry			
C. Can't calm self effectively by sucking on pacifier, looking at toys, or listening to caregiver			
D. Is unable to wait for food or toy without falling apart			
E. Can't change from one activity to another without distress			
F. Demands adult company constantly			
G. Amount of time spent calming child during day (circle one): 15-30 minutes 1-2 hours 3 hours +			
2. Attention			
A. Is easily distractible, shows fleeting attention			
B. Has difficulty paying attention, is difficult to reengage			
C. Is unable to shift focus easily from one object or activity to another			
3. Sleep			
A. Wakes 3 or more times in the night and is unable to fall back to sleep			
B. Requires extensive help to fall asleep; *specify:* rocking, long walks, stroking hair, car ride, other____________			
4. Dressing, Bathing, Touch			
A. Doesn't want to wear clothing			
B. Prefers certain clothing, complains that certain garments are too tight or scratchy			
C. Is distressed by having face or hair washed			
D. Resists cuddling, pulls away or arches			
E. Hates sitting in car seat			
F. Resists being placed in certain positions, such as stomach or back			
G. Is distressed when clothes removed			
5. Movement			
Craves swinging and moving upside-down			

continued

076-1643753-3

Infant/Toddler Symptom Checklist:
13 to18 Months (continued)

	Never or Sometimes	Most Times	Past
6. Listening, Language and Sound			
Startles or is distressed by loud sounds such as vacuum, doorbell, or barking dog			
7. Looking and Sight			
Becomes excited in crowded, bustling settings such as supermarkets, restaurants			
8. Attachment/Emotional Functioning			
A. Avoids eye contact, turns away from the human face, prefers objects and toys			
B. Does not appear happy			
C. Does not initiate interaction with caregiver: Parent needs to woo infant/child constantly			
D. Does not interact reciprocally (back-and-forth exchanges with caregiver)			
E. Has difficulty separating from parents, school, or babysitter			
F. Does not respond at all to limit setting, discipline			
G. Appears anxious or fearful of new people, situations			
H. Needs total control of the environment—"runs the show"			
I. Everyone has difficulty understanding the child's cues or emotions			

How concerned are you about the symptoms checked above? (Circle one.)

Not concerned   Slightly concerned   Moderately concerned   Very concerned

Comments:

Infant/Toddler Symptom Checklist:
13 to 18 Months

Name____ Date_______________

	Never or Sometimes	Most Times	Past
1. Self-Regulation			
A. Is frequently irritable, fussy			
B. Goes easily from whimper to intense cry			
C. Can't calm self effectively by sucking on pacifier, looking at toys, or listening to caregiver			
D. Is unable to wait for food or toy without falling apart			
E. Can't change from one activity to another without distress			
F. Demands adult company constantly			
G. Amount of time spent calming child during day (circle one): 15-30 minutes 1-2 hours 3 hours +			
2. Attention			
A. Is easily distractible, shows fleeting attention			
B. Has difficulty paying attention, is difficult to reengage			
C. Is unable to shift focus easily from one object or activity to another			
3. Sleep			
A. Wakes 3 or more times in the night and is unable to fall back to sleep			
B. Requires extensive help to fall asleep; *specify:* rocking, long walks, stroking hair, car ride, other____________________			
4. Dressing, Bathing, Touch			
A. Doesn't want to wear clothing			
B. Prefers certain clothing, complains that certain garments are too tight or scratchy			
C. Is distressed by having face or hair washed			
D. Resists cuddling, pulls away or arches			
E. Hates sitting in car seat			
F. Resists being placed in certain positions, such as stomach or back			
G. Is distressed when clothes removed			
5. Movement			
Craves swinging and moving upside-down			

continued

076-1643753-3

Infant/Toddler Symptom Checklist: 13 to18 Months (continued)

	Never or Sometimes	Most Times	Past
6. Listening, Language and Sound			
Startles or is distressed by loud sounds such as vacuum, doorbell, or barking dog			
7. Looking and Sight			
Becomes excited in crowded, bustling settings such as supermarkets, restaurants			
8. Attachment/Emotional Functioning			
A. Avoids eye contact, turns away from the human face, prefers objects and toys			
B. Does not appear happy			
C. Does not initiate interaction with caregiver: Parent needs to woo infant/child constantly			
D. Does not interact reciprocally (back-and-forth exchanges with caregiver)			
E. Has difficulty separating from parents, school, or babysitter			
F. Does not respond at all to limit setting, discipline			
G. Appears anxious or fearful of new people, situations			
H. Needs total control of the environment—"runs the show"			
I. Everyone has difficulty understanding the child's cues or emotions			

How concerned are you about the symptoms checked above? (Circle one.)

Not concerned   Slightly concerned   Moderately concerned   Very concerned

Comments:

Infant/Toddler Symptom Checklist:
13 to 18 Months

Name____ Date______________

	Never or Sometimes	Most Times	Past
1. Self-Regulation			
A. Is frequently irritable, fussy			
B. Goes easily from whimper to intense cry			
C. Can't calm self effectively by sucking on pacifier, looking at toys, or listening to caregiver			
D. Is unable to wait for food or toy without falling apart			
E. Can't change from one activity to another without distress			
F. Demands adult company constantly			
G. Amount of time spent calming child during day (circle one): 15-30 minutes 1-2 hours 3 hours +			
2. Attention			
A. Is easily distractible, shows fleeting attention			
B. Has difficulty paying attention, is difficult to reengage			
C. Is unable to shift focus easily from one object or activity to another			
3. Sleep			
A. Wakes 3 or more times in the night and is unable to fall back to sleep			
B. Requires extensive help to fall asleep; *specify:* rocking, long walks, stroking hair, car ride, other____________________			
4. Dressing, Bathing, Touch			
A. Doesn't want to wear clothing			
B. Prefers certain clothing, complains that certain garments are too tight or scratchy			
C. Is distressed by having face or hair washed			
D. Resists cuddling, pulls away or arches			
E. Hates sitting in car seat			
F. Resists being placed in certain positions, such as stomach or back			
G. Is distressed when clothes removed			
5. Movement			
Craves swinging and moving upside-down			

continued

076-1643753-3

Infant/Toddler Symptom Checklist: 13 to18 Months (continued)

	Never or Sometimes	Most Times	Past
6. Listening, Language and Sound			
Startles or is distressed by loud sounds such as vacuum, doorbell, or barking dog			
7. Looking and Sight			
Becomes excited in crowded, bustling settings such as supermarkets, restaurants			
8. Attachment/Emotional Functioning			
A. Avoids eye contact, turns away from the human face, prefers objects and toys			
B. Does not appear happy			
C. Does not initiate interaction with caregiver: Parent needs to woo infant/child constantly			
D. Does not interact reciprocally (back-and-forth exchanges with caregiver)			
E. Has difficulty separating from parents, school, or babysitter			
F. Does not respond at all to limit setting, discipline			
G. Appears anxious or fearful of new people, situations			
H. Needs total control of the environment—"runs the show"			
I. Everyone has difficulty understanding the child's cues or emotions			

How concerned are you about the symptoms checked above? (Circle one.)

Not concerned   Slightly concerned   Moderately concerned   Very concerned

Comments:

Infant/Toddler Symptom Checklist:
13 to 18 Months

Name_______________________________ Date______________

	Never or Sometimes	Most Times	Past
1. Self-Regulation			
A. Is frequently irritable, fussy			
B. Goes easily from whimper to intense cry			
C. Can't calm self effectively by sucking on pacifier, looking at toys, or listening to caregiver			
D. Is unable to wait for food or toy without falling apart			
E. Can't change from one activity to another without distress			
F. Demands adult company constantly			
G. Amount of time spent calming child during day (circle one): 15-30 minutes 1-2 hours 3 hours +			
2. Attention			
A. Is easily distractible, shows fleeting attention			
B. Has difficulty paying attention, is difficult to reengage			
C. Is unable to shift focus easily from one object or activity to another			
3. Sleep			
A. Wakes 3 or more times in the night and is unable to fall back to sleep			
B. Requires extensive help to fall asleep; *specify:* rocking, long walks, stroking hair, car ride, other____________			
4. Dressing, Bathing, Touch			
A. Doesn't want to wear clothing			
B. Prefers certain clothing, complains that certain garments are too tight or scratchy			
C. Is distressed by having face or hair washed			
D. Resists cuddling, pulls away or arches			
E. Hates sitting in car seat			
F. Resists being placed in certain positions, such as stomach or back			
G. Is distressed when clothes removed			
5. Movement			
Craves swinging and moving upside-down			

continued

076-1643753-3

Infant/Toddler Symptom Checklist: 13 to18 Months (continued)

	Never or Sometimes	Most Times	Past
6. Listening, Language and Sound			
Startles or is distressed by loud sounds such as vacuum, doorbell, or barking dog			
7. Looking and Sight			
Becomes excited in crowded, bustling settings such as supermarkets, restaurants			
8. Attachment/Emotional Functioning			
A. Avoids eye contact, turns away from the human face, prefers objects and toys			
B. Does not appear happy			
C. Does not initiate interaction with caregiver: Parent needs to woo infant/child constantly			
D. Does not interact reciprocally (back-and-forth exchanges with caregiver)			
E. Has difficulty separating from parents, school, or babysitter			
F. Does not respond at all to limit setting, discipline			
G. Appears anxious or fearful of new people, situations			
H. Needs total control of the environment—"runs the show"			
I. Everyone has difficulty understanding the child's cues or emotions			

How concerned are you about the symptoms checked above? (Circle one.)

Not concerned   Slightly concerned   Moderately concerned   Very concerned

Comments:

Infant/Toddler Symptom Checklist:
13 to 18 Months

Name______________________________ Date______________

	Never or Sometimes	Most Times	Past
1. Self-Regulation			
A. Is frequently irritable, fussy			
B. Goes easily from whimper to intense cry			
C. Can't calm self effectively by sucking on pacifier, looking at toys, or listening to caregiver			
D. Is unable to wait for food or toy without falling apart			
E. Can't change from one activity to another without distress			
F. Demands adult company constantly			
G. Amount of time spent calming child during day (circle one): 15-30 minutes 1-2 hours 3 hours +			
2. Attention			
A. Is easily distractible, shows fleeting attention			
B. Has difficulty paying attention, is difficult to reengage			
C. Is unable to shift focus easily from one object or activity to another			
3. Sleep			
A. Wakes 3 or more times in the night and is unable to fall back to sleep			
B. Requires extensive help to fall asleep; *specify:* rocking, long walks, stroking hair, car ride, other____________			
4. Dressing, Bathing, Touch			
A. Doesn't want to wear clothing			
B. Prefers certain clothing, complains that certain garments are too tight or scratchy			
C. Is distressed by having face or hair washed			
D. Resists cuddling, pulls away or arches			
E. Hates sitting in car seat			
F. Resists being placed in certain positions, such as stomach or back			
G. Is distressed when clothes removed			
5. Movement			
Craves swinging and moving upside-down			

continued

076-1643753-3

Infant/Toddler Symptom Checklist:
13 to18 Months (continued)

	Never or Sometimes	Most Times	Past
6. Listening, Language and Sound			
Startles or is distressed by loud sounds such as vacuum, doorbell, or barking dog			
7. Looking and Sight			
Becomes excited in crowded, bustling settings such as supermarkets, restaurants			
8. Attachment/Emotional Functioning			
A. Avoids eye contact, turns away from the human face, prefers objects and toys			
B. Does not appear happy			
C. Does not initiate interaction with caregiver: Parent needs to woo infant/child constantly			
D. Does not interact reciprocally (back-and-forth exchanges with caregiver)			
E. Has difficulty separating from parents, school, or babysitter			
F. Does not respond at all to limit setting, discipline			
G. Appears anxious or fearful of new people, situations			
H. Needs total control of the environment—"runs the show"			
I. Everyone has difficulty understanding the child's cues or emotions			

How concerned are you about the symptoms checked above? (Circle one.)

Not concerned Slightly concerned Moderately concerned Very concerned

Comments:

Infant/Toddler Symptom Checklist: 13 to 18 Months

Name________________________________ Date______________

	Never or Sometimes	Most Times	Past
1. Self-Regulation			
A. Is frequently irritable, fussy			
B. Goes easily from whimper to intense cry			
C. Can't calm self effectively by sucking on pacifier, looking at toys, or listening to caregiver			
D. Is unable to wait for food or toy without falling apart			
E. Can't change from one activity to another without distress			
F. Demands adult company constantly			
G. Amount of time spent calming child during day (circle one): 15-30 minutes 1-2 hours 3 hours +			
2. Attention			
A. Is easily distractible, shows fleeting attention			
B. Has difficulty paying attention, is difficult to reengage			
C. Is unable to shift focus easily from one object or activity to another			
3. Sleep			
A. Wakes 3 or more times in the night and is unable to fall back to sleep			
B. Requires extensive help to fall asleep; *specify:* rocking, long walks, stroking hair, car ride, other__________			
4. Dressing, Bathing, Touch			
A. Doesn't want to wear clothing			
B. Prefers certain clothing, complains that certain garments are too tight or scratchy			
C. Is distressed by having face or hair washed			
D. Resists cuddling, pulls away or arches			
E. Hates sitting in car seat			
F. Resists being placed in certain positions, such as stomach or back			
G. Is distressed when clothes removed			
5. Movement			
Craves swinging and moving upside-down			

continued

076-1643753-3

Infant/Toddler Symptom Checklist:
13 to18 Months (continued)

	Never or Sometimes	Most Times	Past
6. Listening, Language and Sound			
Startles or is distressed by loud sounds such as vacuum, doorbell, or barking dog			
7. Looking and Sight			
Becomes excited in crowded, bustling settings such as supermarkets, restaurants			
8. Attachment/Emotional Functioning			
A. Avoids eye contact, turns away from the human face, prefers objects and toys			
B. Does not appear happy			
C. Does not initiate interaction with caregiver: Parent needs to woo infant/child constantly			
D. Does not interact reciprocally (back-and-forth exchanges with caregiver)			
E. Has difficulty separating from parents, school, or babysitter			
F. Does not respond at all to limit setting, discipline			
G. Appears anxious or fearful of new people, situations			
H. Needs total control of the environment—"runs the show"			
I. Everyone has difficulty understanding the child's cues or emotions			

How concerned are you about the symptoms checked above? (Circle one.)

Not concerned Slightly concerned Moderately concerned Very concerned

Comments:

Infant/Toddler Symptom Checklist:
13 to 18 Months

Name________________________________ Date______________

	Never or Sometimes	Most Times	Past
1. Self-Regulation			
A. Is frequently irritable, fussy			
B. Goes easily from whimper to intense cry			
C. Can't calm self effectively by sucking on pacifier, looking at toys, or listening to caregiver			
D. Is unable to wait for food or toy without falling apart			
E. Can't change from one activity to another without distress			
F. Demands adult company constantly			
G. Amount of time spent calming child during day (circle one): 15-30 minutes 1-2 hours 3 hours +			
2. Attention			
A. Is easily distractible, shows fleeting attention			
B. Has difficulty paying attention, is difficult to reengage			
C. Is unable to shift focus easily from one object or activity to another			
3. Sleep			
A. Wakes 3 or more times in the night and is unable to fall back to sleep			
B. Requires extensive help to fall asleep; *specify:* rocking, long walks, stroking hair, car ride, other__________			
4. Dressing, Bathing, Touch			
A. Doesn't want to wear clothing			
B. Prefers certain clothing, complains that certain garments are too tight or scratchy			
C. Is distressed by having face or hair washed			
D. Resists cuddling, pulls away or arches			
E. Hates sitting in car seat			
F. Resists being placed in certain positions, such as stomach or back			
G. Is distressed when clothes removed			
5. Movement			
Craves swinging and moving upside-down			

continued

076-1643753-3

Infant/Toddler Symptom Checklist:
13 to18 Months (continued)

	Never or Sometimes	Most Times	Past
6. Listening, Language and Sound			
Startles or is distressed by loud sounds such as vacuum, doorbell, or barking dog			
7. Looking and Sight			
Becomes excited in crowded, bustling settings such as supermarkets, restaurants			
8. Attachment/Emotional Functioning			
A. Avoids eye contact, turns away from the human face, prefers objects and toys			
B. Does not appear happy			
C. Does not initiate interaction with caregiver: Parent needs to woo infant/child constantly			
D. Does not interact reciprocally (back-and-forth exchanges with caregiver)			
E. Has difficulty separating from parents, school, or babysitter			
F. Does not respond at all to limit setting, discipline			
G. Appears anxious or fearful of new people, situations			
H. Needs total control of the environment—"runs the show"			
I. Everyone has difficulty understanding the child's cues or emotions			

How concerned are you about the symptoms checked above? (Circle one.)

Not concerned Slightly concerned Moderately concerned Very concerned

Comments:

Infant/Toddler Symptom Checklist:
13 to 18 Months

Name________________________________ Date______________

	Never or Sometimes	Most Times	Past
1. Self-Regulation			
A. Is frequently irritable, fussy			
B. Goes easily from whimper to intense cry			
C. Can't calm self effectively by sucking on pacifier, looking at toys, or listening to caregiver			
D. Is unable to wait for food or toy without falling apart			
E. Can't change from one activity to another without distress			
F. Demands adult company constantly			
G. Amount of time spent calming child during day (circle one): 15-30 minutes 1-2 hours 3 hours +			
2. Attention			
A. Is easily distractible, shows fleeting attention			
B. Has difficulty paying attention, is difficult to reengage			
C. Is unable to shift focus easily from one object or activity to another			
3. Sleep			
A. Wakes 3 or more times in the night and is unable to fall back to sleep			
B. Requires extensive help to fall asleep; *specify:* rocking, long walks, stroking hair, car ride, other______________			
4. Dressing, Bathing, Touch			
A. Doesn't want to wear clothing			
B. Prefers certain clothing, complains that certain garments are too tight or scratchy			
C. Is distressed by having face or hair washed			
D. Resists cuddling, pulls away or arches			
E. Hates sitting in car seat			
F. Resists being placed in certain positions, such as stomach or back			
G. Is distressed when clothes removed			
5. Movement			
Craves swinging and moving upside-down			

continued

076-1643753-3

Infant/Toddler Symptom Checklist:
13 to18 Months (continued)

	Never or Sometimes	Most Times	Past
6. Listening, Language and Sound			
Startles or is distressed by loud sounds such as vacuum, doorbell, or barking dog			
7. Looking and Sight			
Becomes excited in crowded, bustling settings such as supermarkets, restaurants			
8. Attachment/Emotional Functioning			
A. Avoids eye contact, turns away from the human face, prefers objects and toys			
B. Does not appear happy			
C. Does not initiate interaction with caregiver: Parent needs to woo infant/child constantly			
D. Does not interact reciprocally (back-and-forth exchanges with caregiver)			
E. Has difficulty separating from parents, school, or babysitter			
F. Does not respond at all to limit setting, discipline			
G. Appears anxious or fearful of new people, situations			
H. Needs total control of the environment—"runs the show"			
I. Everyone has difficulty understanding the child's cues or emotions			

How concerned are you about the symptoms checked above? (Circle one.)

Not concerned   Slightly concerned   Moderately concerned   Very concerned

Comments:

Infant/Toddler Symptom Checklist:
13 to 18 Months

Name____ Date______________

	Never or Sometimes	Most Times	Past
1. Self-Regulation			
A. Is frequently irritable, fussy			
B. Goes easily from whimper to intense cry			
C. Can't calm self effectively by sucking on pacifier, looking at toys, or listening to caregiver			
D. Is unable to wait for food or toy without falling apart			
E. Can't change from one activity to another without distress			
F. Demands adult company constantly			
G. Amount of time spent calming child during day (circle one): 15-30 minutes 1-2 hours 3 hours +			
2. Attention			
A. Is easily distractible, shows fleeting attention			
B. Has difficulty paying attention, is difficult to reengage			
C. Is unable to shift focus easily from one object or activity to another			
3. Sleep			
A. Wakes 3 or more times in the night and is unable to fall back to sleep			
B. Requires extensive help to fall asleep; *specify:* rocking, long walks, stroking hair, car ride, other____________________			
4. Dressing, Bathing, Touch			
A. Doesn't want to wear clothing			
B. Prefers certain clothing, complains that certain garments are too tight or scratchy			
C. Is distressed by having face or hair washed			
D. Resists cuddling, pulls away or arches			
E. Hates sitting in car seat			
F. Resists being placed in certain positions, such as stomach or back			
G. Is distressed when clothes removed			
5. Movement			
Craves swinging and moving upside-down			

continued

076-1643753-3

Infant/Toddler Symptom Checklist:
13 to18 Months (continued)

	Never or Sometimes	Most Times	Past
6. Listening, Language and Sound			
Startles or is distressed by loud sounds such as vacuum, doorbell, or barking dog			
7. Looking and Sight			
Becomes excited in crowded, bustling settings such as supermarkets, restaurants			
8. Attachment/Emotional Functioning			
A. Avoids eye contact, turns away from the human face, prefers objects and toys			
B. Does not appear happy			
C. Does not initiate interaction with caregiver: Parent needs to woo infant/child constantly			
D. Does not interact reciprocally (back-and-forth exchanges with caregiver)			
E. Has difficulty separating from parents, school, or babysitter			
F. Does not respond at all to limit setting, discipline			
G. Appears anxious or fearful of new people, situations			
H. Needs total control of the environment—"runs the show"			
I. Everyone has difficulty understanding the child's cues or emotions			

How concerned are you about the symptoms checked above? (Circle one.)

Not concerned Slightly concerned Moderately concerned Very concerned

Comments:

Infant/Toddler Symptom Checklist:
19 to 24 Months

Name______________________________ Date______________

	Never or Sometimes	Most Times	Past
1. Self-Regulation			
A. Goes easily from whimper to intense cry			
B. Can't calm self effectively by sucking on pacifier, looking at toys, or listening to caregiver			
C. Is unable to wait for food or toy without falling apart			
D. Must be prepared several times in advance before change is introduced			
E. Demands adult company constantly			
2. Attention			
A. Is easily distractible, shows fleeting attention			
B. Has difficulty paying attention, is difficult to reengage			
3. Sleep			
Wakes 3 or more times in the night and is unable to fall back to sleep			
4. Eating or Feeding			
A. Craves certain foods or drinks			
B. Is too distracted to stay seated for meals			
5. Dressing, Bathing, Touch			
A. Resists cuddling, pulls away or arches			
B. Hates sitting in car seat			
C. Resists being placed in certain positions, such as stomach or back			
6. Movement			
A. Is in constant movement—rocking, running about, unable to sit still for an activity			
B. Craves swinging and moving upside-down			
C. Is clumsy—falls, has poor balance, bumps into things			
7. Listening, Language and Sound			
A. Is distracted by sounds the average person doesn't notice			
B. Doesn't respond to verbal cues (hearing not a problem)			
C. Repeats or echoes previously heard words, phrases, or sentences			

continued

Infant/Toddler Symptom Checklist: 19 to 24 Months (continued)

	Never or Sometimes	Most Times	Past
8. Looking and Sight			
Becomes excited in crowded, bustling settings such as supermarkets, restaurants			
9. Attachment/Emotional Functioning			
A. Does not play with other children—withdraws or is aggressive			
B. Does not respond at all to limits, discipline			
C. Needs total control of the environment—"runs the show"			

How concerned are you about the symptoms checked above? (Circle one.)

Not concerned   Slightly concerned   Moderately concerned   Very concerned

Comments:

Infant/Toddler Symptom Checklist:
19 to 24 Months

Name________________________ Date____________

	Never or Sometimes	Most Times	Past
1. Self-Regulation			
A. Goes easily from whimper to intense cry			
B. Can't calm self effectively by sucking on pacifier, looking at toys, or listening to caregiver			
C. Is unable to wait for food or toy without falling apart			
D. Must be prepared several times in advance before change is introduced			
E. Demands adult company constantly			
2. Attention			
A. Is easily distractible, shows fleeting attention			
B. Has difficulty paying attention, is difficult to reengage			
3. Sleep			
Wakes 3 or more times in the night and is unable to fall back to sleep			
4. Eating or Feeding			
A. Craves certain foods or drinks			
B. Is too distracted to stay seated for meals			
5. Dressing, Bathing, Touch			
A. Resists cuddling, pulls away or arches			
B. Hates sitting in car seat			
C. Resists being placed in certain positions, such as stomach or back			
6. Movement			
A. Is in constant movement—rocking, running about, unable to sit still for an activity			
B. Craves swinging and moving upside-down			
C. Is clumsy—falls, has poor balance, bumps into things			
7. Listening, Language and Sound			
A. Is distracted by sounds the average person doesn't notice			
B. Doesn't respond to verbal cues (hearing not a problem)			
C. Repeats or echoes previously heard words, phrases, or sentences			

continued

076-1643753-4

Infant/Toddler Symptom Checklist: 19 to 24 Months (continued)

	Never or Sometimes	Most Times	Past
8. Looking and Sight			
Becomes excited in crowded, bustling settings such as supermarkets, restaurants			
9. Attachment/Emotional Functioning			
A. Does not play with other children—withdraws or is aggressive			
B. Does not respond at all to limits, discipline			
C. Needs total control of the environment—"runs the show"			

How concerned are you about the symptoms checked above? (Circle one.)

Not concerned Slightly concerned Moderately concerned Very concerned

Comments:

Infant/Toddler Symptom Checklist: 19 to 24 Months

Name______________________________ Date______________

	Never or Sometimes	Most Times	Past
1. Self-Regulation			
A. Goes easily from whimper to intense cry			
B. Can't calm self effectively by sucking on pacifier, looking at toys, or listening to caregiver			
C. Is unable to wait for food or toy without falling apart			
D. Must be prepared several times in advance before change is introduced			
E. Demands adult company constantly			
2. Attention			
A. Is easily distractible, shows fleeting attention			
B. Has difficulty paying attention, is difficult to reengage			
3. Sleep			
Wakes 3 or more times in the night and is unable to fall back to sleep			
4. Eating or Feeding			
A. Craves certain foods or drinks			
B. Is too distracted to stay seated for meals			
5. Dressing, Bathing, Touch			
A. Resists cuddling, pulls away or arches			
B. Hates sitting in car seat			
C. Resists being placed in certain positions, such as stomach or back			
6. Movement			
A. Is in constant movement—rocking, running about, unable to sit still for an activity			
B. Craves swinging and moving upside-down			
C. Is clumsy—falls, has poor balance, bumps into things			
7. Listening, Language and Sound			
A. Is distracted by sounds the average person doesn't notice			
B. Doesn't respond to verbal cues (hearing not a problem)			
C. Repeats or echoes previously heard words, phrases, or sentences			

continued

076-1643753-4

Infant/Toddler Symptom Checklist:
19 to 24 Months (continued)

	Never or Sometimes	Most Times	Past
8. Looking and Sight			
Becomes excited in crowded, bustling settings such as supermarkets, restaurants			
9. Attachment/Emotional Functioning			
A. Does not play with other children—withdraws or is aggressive			
B. Does not respond at all to limits, discipline			
C. Needs total control of the environment—"runs the show"			

How concerned are you about the symptoms checked above? (Circle one.)

Not concerned   Slightly concerned   Moderately concerned   Very concerned

Comments:

Infant/Toddler Symptom Checklist: 19 to 24 Months

Name________________________________ Date______________

	Never or Sometimes	Most Times	Past
1. Self-Regulation			
A. Goes easily from whimper to intense cry			
B. Can't calm self effectively by sucking on pacifier, looking at toys, or listening to caregiver			
C. Is unable to wait for food or toy without falling apart			
D. Must be prepared several times in advance before change is introduced			
E. Demands adult company constantly			
2. Attention			
A. Is easily distractible, shows fleeting attention			
B. Has difficulty paying attention, is difficult to reengage			
3. Sleep			
Wakes 3 or more times in the night and is unable to fall back to sleep			
4. Eating or Feeding			
A. Craves certain foods or drinks			
B. Is too distracted to stay seated for meals			
5. Dressing, Bathing, Touch			
A. Resists cuddling, pulls away or arches			
B. Hates sitting in car seat			
C. Resists being placed in certain positions, such as stomach or back			
6. Movement			
A. Is in constant movement—rocking, running about, unable to sit still for an activity			
B. Craves swinging and moving upside-down			
C. Is clumsy—falls, has poor balance, bumps into things			
7. Listening, Language and Sound			
A. Is distracted by sounds the average person doesn't notice			
B. Doesn't respond to verbal cues (hearing not a problem)			
C. Repeats or echoes previously heard words, phrases, or sentences			

continued

076-1643753-4

Infant/Toddler Symptom Checklist: 19 to 24 Months (continued)

	Never or Sometimes	Most Times	Past
8. Looking and Sight			
Becomes excited in crowded, bustling settings such as supermarkets, restaurants			
9. Attachment/Emotional Functioning			
A. Does not play with other children—withdraws or is aggressive			
B. Does not respond at all to limits, discipline			
C. Needs total control of the environment—"runs the show"			

How concerned are you about the symptoms checked above? (Circle one.)

Not concerned   Slightly concerned   Moderately concerned   Very concerned

Comments:

Infant/Toddler Symptom Checklist: 19 to 24 Months

Name________________________ Date______________

	Never or Sometimes	Most Times	Past
1. Self-Regulation			
A. Goes easily from whimper to intense cry			
B. Can't calm self effectively by sucking on pacifier, looking at toys, or listening to caregiver			
C. Is unable to wait for food or toy without falling apart			
D. Must be prepared several times in advance before change is introduced			
E. Demands adult company constantly			
2. Attention			
A. Is easily distractible, shows fleeting attention			
B. Has difficulty paying attention, is difficult to reengage			
3. Sleep			
Wakes 3 or more times in the night and is unable to fall back to sleep			
4. Eating or Feeding			
A. Craves certain foods or drinks			
B. Is too distracted to stay seated for meals			
5. Dressing, Bathing, Touch			
A. Resists cuddling, pulls away or arches			
B. Hates sitting in car seat			
C. Resists being placed in certain positions, such as stomach or back			
6. Movement			
A. Is in constant movement—rocking, running about, unable to sit still for an activity			
B. Craves swinging and moving upside-down			
C. Is clumsy—falls, has poor balance, bumps into things			
7. Listening, Language and Sound			
A. Is distracted by sounds the average person doesn't notice			
B. Doesn't respond to verbal cues (hearing not a problem)			
C. Repeats or echoes previously heard words, phrases, or sentences			

continued

076-1643753-4

Infant/Toddler Symptom Checklist:
19 to 24 Months (continued)

	Never or Sometimes	Most Times	Past
8. Looking and Sight			
Becomes excited in crowded, bustling settings such as supermarkets, restaurants			
9. Attachment/Emotional Functioning			
A. Does not play with other children—withdraws or is aggressive			
B. Does not respond at all to limits, discipline			
C. Needs total control of the environment—"runs the show"			

How concerned are you about the symptoms checked above? (Circle one.)

Not concerned Slightly concerned Moderately concerned Very concerned

Comments:

Infant/Toddler Symptom Checklist:
19 to 24 Months

Name________________________ Date______________

	Never or Sometimes	Most Times	Past
1. Self-Regulation			
A. Goes easily from whimper to intense cry			
B. Can't calm self effectively by sucking on pacifier, looking at toys, or listening to caregiver			
C. Is unable to wait for food or toy without falling apart			
D. Must be prepared several times in advance before change is introduced			
E. Demands adult company constantly			
2. Attention			
A. Is easily distractible, shows fleeting attention			
B. Has difficulty paying attention, is difficult to reengage			
3. Sleep			
Wakes 3 or more times in the night and is unable to fall back to sleep			
4. Eating or Feeding			
A. Craves certain foods or drinks			
B. Is too distracted to stay seated for meals			
5. Dressing, Bathing, Touch			
A. Resists cuddling, pulls away or arches			
B. Hates sitting in car seat			
C. Resists being placed in certain positions, such as stomach or back			
6. Movement			
A. Is in constant movement—rocking, running about, unable to sit still for an activity			
B. Craves swinging and moving upside-down			
C. Is clumsy—falls, has poor balance, bumps into things			
7. Listening, Language and Sound			
A. Is distracted by sounds the average person doesn't notice			
B. Doesn't respond to verbal cues (hearing not a problem)			
C. Repeats or echoes previously heard words, phrases, or sentences			

continued

076-1643753-4

Infant/Toddler Symptom Checklist:
19 to 24 Months (continued)

	Never or Sometimes	Most Times	Past
8. Looking and Sight			
Becomes excited in crowded, bustling settings such as supermarkets, restaurants			
9. Attachment/Emotional Functioning			
A. Does not play with other children—withdraws or is aggressive			
B. Does not respond at all to limits, discipline			
C. Needs total control of the environment—"runs the show"			

How concerned are you about the symptoms checked above? (Circle one.)

Not concerned   Slightly concerned   Moderately concerned   Very concerned

Comments:

Infant/Toddler Symptom Checklist: 19 to 24 Months

Name______________________________ Date______________

	Never or Sometimes	Most Times	Past
1. Self-Regulation			
A. Goes easily from whimper to intense cry			
B. Can't calm self effectively by sucking on pacifier, looking at toys, or listening to caregiver			
C. Is unable to wait for food or toy without falling apart			
D. Must be prepared several times in advance before change is introduced			
E. Demands adult company constantly			
2. Attention			
A. Is easily distractible, shows fleeting attention			
B. Has difficulty paying attention, is difficult to reengage			
3. Sleep			
Wakes 3 or more times in the night and is unable to fall back to sleep			
4. Eating or Feeding			
A. Craves certain foods or drinks			
B. Is too distracted to stay seated for meals			
5. Dressing, Bathing, Touch			
A. Resists cuddling, pulls away or arches			
B. Hates sitting in car seat			
C. Resists being placed in certain positions, such as stomach or back			
6. Movement			
A. Is in constant movement—rocking, running about, unable to sit still for an activity			
B. Craves swinging and moving upside-down			
C. Is clumsy—falls, has poor balance, bumps into things			
7. Listening, Language and Sound			
A. Is distracted by sounds the average person doesn't notice			
B. Doesn't respond to verbal cues (hearing not a problem)			
C. Repeats or echoes previously heard words, phrases, or sentences			

continued

076-1643753-4

Infant/Toddler Symptom Checklist:
19 to 24 Months (continued)

	Never or Sometimes	Most Times	Past
8. Looking and Sight			
Becomes excited in crowded, bustling settings such as supermarkets, restaurants			
9. Attachment/Emotional Functioning			
A. Does not play with other children—withdraws or is aggressive			
B. Does not respond at all to limits, discipline			
C. Needs total control of the environment—"runs the show"			

How concerned are you about the symptoms checked above? (Circle one.)

Not concerned   Slightly concerned   Moderately concerned   Very concerned

Comments:

Infant/Toddler Symptom Checklist:
19 to 24 Months

Name______________________ Date__________

	Never or Sometimes	Most Times	Past
1. Self-Regulation			
A. Goes easily from whimper to intense cry			
B. Can't calm self effectively by sucking on pacifier, looking at toys, or listening to caregiver			
C. Is unable to wait for food or toy without falling apart			
D. Must be prepared several times in advance before change is introduced			
E. Demands adult company constantly			
2. Attention			
A. Is easily distractible, shows fleeting attention			
B. Has difficulty paying attention, is difficult to reengage			
3. Sleep			
Wakes 3 or more times in the night and is unable to fall back to sleep			
4. Eating or Feeding			
A. Craves certain foods or drinks			
B. Is too distracted to stay seated for meals			
5. Dressing, Bathing, Touch			
A. Resists cuddling, pulls away or arches			
B. Hates sitting in car seat			
C. Resists being placed in certain positions, such as stomach or back			
6. Movement			
A. Is in constant movement—rocking, running about, unable to sit still for an activity			
B. Craves swinging and moving upside-down			
C. Is clumsy—falls, has poor balance, bumps into things			
7. Listening, Language and Sound			
A. Is distracted by sounds the average person doesn't notice			
B. Doesn't respond to verbal cues (hearing not a problem)			
C. Repeats or echoes previously heard words, phrases, or sentences			

continued

Infant/Toddler Symptom Checklist:
19 to 24 Months (continued)

	Never or Sometimes	Most Times	Past
8. Looking and Sight			
Becomes excited in crowded, bustling settings such as supermarkets, restaurants			
9. Attachment/Emotional Functioning			
A. Does not play with other children—withdraws or is aggressive			
B. Does not respond at all to limits, discipline			
C. Needs total control of the environment—"runs the show"			

How concerned are you about the symptoms checked above? (Circle one.)

Not concerned   Slightly concerned   Moderately concerned   Very concerned

Comments:

Infant/Toddler Symptom Checklist:
19 to 24 Months

Name______________________________ Date______________

	Never or Sometimes	Most Times	Past
1. Self-Regulation			
A. Goes easily from whimper to intense cry			
B. Can't calm self effectively by sucking on pacifier, looking at toys, or listening to caregiver			
C. Is unable to wait for food or toy without falling apart			
D. Must be prepared several times in advance before change is introduced			
E. Demands adult company constantly			
2. Attention			
A. Is easily distractible, shows fleeting attention			
B. Has difficulty paying attention, is difficult to reengage			
3. Sleep			
Wakes 3 or more times in the night and is unable to fall back to sleep			
4. Eating or Feeding			
A. Craves certain foods or drinks			
B. Is too distracted to stay seated for meals			
5. Dressing, Bathing, Touch			
A. Resists cuddling, pulls away or arches			
B. Hates sitting in car seat			
C. Resists being placed in certain positions, such as stomach or back			
6. Movement			
A. Is in constant movement—rocking, running about, unable to sit still for an activity			
B. Craves swinging and moving upside-down			
C. Is clumsy—falls, has poor balance, bumps into things			
7. Listening, Language and Sound			
A. Is distracted by sounds the average person doesn't notice			
B. Doesn't respond to verbal cues (hearing not a problem)			
C. Repeats or echoes previously heard words, phrases, or sentences			

continued

076-1643753-4

Infant/Toddler Symptom Checklist:
19 to 24 Months (continued)

	Never or Sometimes	Most Times	Past
8. Looking and Sight			
Becomes excited in crowded, bustling settings such as supermarkets, restaurants			
9. Attachment/Emotional Functioning			
A. Does not play with other children—withdraws or is aggressive			
B. Does not respond at all to limits, discipline			
C. Needs total control of the environment—"runs the show"			

How concerned are you about the symptoms checked above? (Circle one.)

Not concerned   Slightly concerned   Moderately concerned   Very concerned

Comments:

Infant/Toddler Symptom Checklist:
19 to 24 Months

Name________________________________ Date______________

	Never or Sometimes	Most Times	Past
1. Self-Regulation			
A. Goes easily from whimper to intense cry			
B. Can't calm self effectively by sucking on pacifier, looking at toys, or listening to caregiver			
C. Is unable to wait for food or toy without falling apart			
D. Must be prepared several times in advance before change is introduced			
E. Demands adult company constantly			
2. Attention			
A. Is easily distractible, shows fleeting attention			
B. Has difficulty paying attention, is difficult to reengage			
3. Sleep			
Wakes 3 or more times in the night and is unable to fall back to sleep			
4. Eating or Feeding			
A. Craves certain foods or drinks			
B. Is too distracted to stay seated for meals			
5. Dressing, Bathing, Touch			
A. Resists cuddling, pulls away or arches			
B. Hates sitting in car seat			
C. Resists being placed in certain positions, such as stomach or back			
6. Movement			
A. Is in constant movement—rocking, running about, unable to sit still for an activity			
B. Craves swinging and moving upside-down			
C. Is clumsy—falls, has poor balance, bumps into things			
7. Listening, Language and Sound			
A. Is distracted by sounds the average person doesn't notice			
B. Doesn't respond to verbal cues (hearing not a problem)			
C. Repeats or echoes previously heard words, phrases, or sentences			

continued

076-1643753-4

Infant/Toddler Symptom Checklist:
19 to 24 Months (continued)

	Never or Sometimes	Most Times	Past
8. Looking and Sight			
Becomes excited in crowded, bustling settings such as supermarkets, restaurants			
9. Attachment/Emotional Functioning			
A. Does not play with other children—withdraws or is aggressive			
B. Does not respond at all to limits, discipline			
C. Needs total control of the environment—"runs the show"			

How concerned are you about the symptoms checked above? (Circle one.)

Not concerned   Slightly concerned   Moderately concerned   Very concerned

Comments:

Infant/Toddler Symptom Checklist:
19 to 24 Months

Name____ Date________________

	Never or Sometimes	Most Times	Past
1. Self-Regulation			
A. Goes easily from whimper to intense cry			
B. Can't calm self effectively by sucking on pacifier, looking at toys, or listening to caregiver			
C. Is unable to wait for food or toy without falling apart			
D. Must be prepared several times in advance before change is introduced			
E. Demands adult company constantly			
2. Attention			
A. Is easily distractible, shows fleeting attention			
B. Has difficulty paying attention, is difficult to reengage			
3. Sleep			
Wakes 3 or more times in the night and is unable to fall back to sleep			
4. Eating or Feeding			
A. Craves certain foods or drinks			
B. Is too distracted to stay seated for meals			
5. Dressing, Bathing, Touch			
A. Resists cuddling, pulls away or arches			
B. Hates sitting in car seat			
C. Resists being placed in certain positions, such as stomach or back			
6. Movement			
A. Is in constant movement—rocking, running about, unable to sit still for an activity			
B. Craves swinging and moving upside-down			
C. Is clumsy—falls, has poor balance, bumps into things			
7. Listening, Language and Sound			
A. Is distracted by sounds the average person doesn't notice			
B. Doesn't respond to verbal cues (hearing not a problem)			
C. Repeats or echoes previously heard words, phrases, or sentences			

continued

Infant/Toddler Symptom Checklist:
19 to 24 Months (continued)

	Never or Sometimes	Most Times	Past
8. Looking and Sight			
Becomes excited in crowded, bustling settings such as supermarkets, restaurants			
9. Attachment/Emotional Functioning			
A. Does not play with other children—withdraws or is aggressive			
B. Does not respond at all to limits, discipline			
C. Needs total control of the environment—"runs the show"			

How concerned are you about the symptoms checked above? (Circle one.)

Not concerned   Slightly concerned   Moderately concerned   Very concerned

Comments:

Infant/Toddler Symptom Checklist:
19 to 24 Months

Name____ Date______________

	Never or Sometimes	Most Times	Past
1. Self-Regulation			
A. Goes easily from whimper to intense cry			
B. Can't calm self effectively by sucking on pacifier, looking at toys, or listening to caregiver			
C. Is unable to wait for food or toy without falling apart			
D. Must be prepared several times in advance before change is introduced			
E. Demands adult company constantly			
2. Attention			
A. Is easily distractible, shows fleeting attention			
B. Has difficulty paying attention, is difficult to reengage			
3. Sleep			
Wakes 3 or more times in the night and is unable to fall back to sleep			
4. Eating or Feeding			
A. Craves certain foods or drinks			
B. Is too distracted to stay seated for meals			
5. Dressing, Bathing, Touch			
A. Resists cuddling, pulls away or arches			
B. Hates sitting in car seat			
C. Resists being placed in certain positions, such as stomach or back			
6. Movement			
A. Is in constant movement—rocking, running about, unable to sit still for an activity			
B. Craves swinging and moving upside-down			
C. Is clumsy—falls, has poor balance, bumps into things			
7. Listening, Language and Sound			
A. Is distracted by sounds the average person doesn't notice			
B. Doesn't respond to verbal cues (hearing not a problem)			
C. Repeats or echoes previously heard words, phrases, or sentences			

continued

076-1643753-4

Infant/Toddler Symptom Checklist: 19 to 24 Months (continued)

	Never or Sometimes	Most Times	Past
8. Looking and Sight			
Becomes excited in crowded, bustling settings such as supermarkets, restaurants			
9. Attachment/Emotional Functioning			
A. Does not play with other children—withdraws or is aggressive			
B. Does not respond at all to limits, discipline			
C. Needs total control of the environment—"runs the show"			

How concerned are you about the symptoms checked above? (Circle one.)

Not concerned Slightly concerned Moderately concerned Very concerned

Comments:

Infant/Toddler Symptom Checklist: 19 to 24 Months

Name______________________________ Date______________

	Never or Sometimes	Most Times	Past
1. Self-Regulation			
A. Goes easily from whimper to intense cry			
B. Can't calm self effectively by sucking on pacifier, looking at toys, or listening to caregiver			
C. Is unable to wait for food or toy without falling apart			
D. Must be prepared several times in advance before change is introduced			
E. Demands adult company constantly			
2. Attention			
A. Is easily distractible, shows fleeting attention			
B. Has difficulty paying attention, is difficult to reengage			
3. Sleep			
Wakes 3 or more times in the night and is unable to fall back to sleep			
4. Eating or Feeding			
A. Craves certain foods or drinks			
B. Is too distracted to stay seated for meals			
5. Dressing, Bathing, Touch			
A. Resists cuddling, pulls away or arches			
B. Hates sitting in car seat			
C. Resists being placed in certain positions, such as stomach or back			
6. Movement			
A. Is in constant movement—rocking, running about, unable to sit still for an activity			
B. Craves swinging and moving upside-down			
C. Is clumsy—falls, has poor balance, bumps into things			
7. Listening, Language and Sound			
A. Is distracted by sounds the average person doesn't notice			
B. Doesn't respond to verbal cues (hearing not a problem)			
C. Repeats or echoes previously heard words, phrases, or sentences			

continued

076-1643753-4

Infant/Toddler Symptom Checklist:
19 to 24 Months (continued)

	Never or Sometimes	Most Times	Past
8. Looking and Sight			
Becomes excited in crowded, bustling settings such as supermarkets, restaurants			
9. Attachment/Emotional Functioning			
A. Does not play with other children—withdraws or is aggressive			
B. Does not respond at all to limits, discipline			
C. Needs total control of the environment—"runs the show"			

How concerned are you about the symptoms checked above? (Circle one.)

Not concerned Slightly concerned Moderately concerned Very concerned

Comments:

Infant/Toddler Symptom Checklist:
19 to 24 Months

Name________________________________ Date______________

	Never or Sometimes	Most Times	Past
1. Self-Regulation			
A. Goes easily from whimper to intense cry			
B. Can't calm self effectively by sucking on pacifier, looking at toys, or listening to caregiver			
C. Is unable to wait for food or toy without falling apart			
D. Must be prepared several times in advance before change is introduced			
E. Demands adult company constantly			
2. Attention			
A. Is easily distractible, shows fleeting attention			
B. Has difficulty paying attention, is difficult to reengage			
3. Sleep			
Wakes 3 or more times in the night and is unable to fall back to sleep			
4. Eating or Feeding			
A. Craves certain foods or drinks			
B. Is too distracted to stay seated for meals			
5. Dressing, Bathing, Touch			
A. Resists cuddling, pulls away or arches			
B. Hates sitting in car seat			
C. Resists being placed in certain positions, such as stomach or back			
6. Movement			
A. Is in constant movement—rocking, running about, unable to sit still for an activity			
B. Craves swinging and moving upside-down			
C. Is clumsy—falls, has poor balance, bumps into things			
7. Listening, Language and Sound			
A. Is distracted by sounds the average person doesn't notice			
B. Doesn't respond to verbal cues (hearing not a problem)			
C. Repeats or echoes previously heard words, phrases, or sentences			

continued

076-1643753-4

Infant/Toddler Symptom Checklist:
19 to 24 Months (continued)

	Never or Sometimes	Most Times	Past
8. Looking and Sight			
Becomes excited in crowded, bustling settings such as supermarkets, restaurants			
9. Attachment/Emotional Functioning			
A. Does not play with other children—withdraws or is aggressive			
B. Does not respond at all to limits, discipline			
C. Needs total control of the environment—"runs the show"			

How concerned are you about the symptoms checked above? (Circle one.)

Not concerned   Slightly concerned   Moderately concerned   Very concerned

Comments:

Infant/Toddler Symptom Checklist: 19 to 24 Months

Name________________________ Date____________

	Never or Sometimes	Most Times	Past
1. Self-Regulation			
A. Goes easily from whimper to intense cry			
B. Can't calm self effectively by sucking on pacifier, looking at toys, or listening to caregiver			
C. Is unable to wait for food or toy without falling apart			
D. Must be prepared several times in advance before change is introduced			
E. Demands adult company constantly			
2. Attention			
A. Is easily distractible, shows fleeting attention			
B. Has difficulty paying attention, is difficult to reengage			
3. Sleep			
Wakes 3 or more times in the night and is unable to fall back to sleep			
4. Eating or Feeding			
A. Craves certain foods or drinks			
B. Is too distracted to stay seated for meals			
5. Dressing, Bathing, Touch			
A. Resists cuddling, pulls away or arches			
B. Hates sitting in car seat			
C. Resists being placed in certain positions, such as stomach or back			
6. Movement			
A. Is in constant movement—rocking, running about, unable to sit still for an activity			
B. Craves swinging and moving upside-down			
C. Is clumsy—falls, has poor balance, bumps into things			
7. Listening, Language and Sound			
A. Is distracted by sounds the average person doesn't notice			
B. Doesn't respond to verbal cues (hearing not a problem)			
C. Repeats or echoes previously heard words, phrases, or sentences			

continued

076-1643753-4

Infant/Toddler Symptom Checklist:
19 to 24 Months (continued)

	Never or Sometimes	Most Times	Past
8. Looking and Sight			
Becomes excited in crowded, bustling settings such as supermarkets, restaurants			
9. Attachment/Emotional Functioning			
A. Does not play with other children—withdraws or is aggressive			
B. Does not respond at all to limits, discipline			
C. Needs total control of the environment—"runs the show"			

How concerned are you about the symptoms checked above? (Circle one.)

Not concerned　　Slightly concerned　　Moderately concerned　　Very concerned

Comments:

Infant/Toddler Symptom Checklist:
19 to 24 Months

Name________________________________ Date______________

	Never or Sometimes	Most Times	Past
1. Self-Regulation			
A. Goes easily from whimper to intense cry			
B. Can't calm self effectively by sucking on pacifier, looking at toys, or listening to caregiver			
C. Is unable to wait for food or toy without falling apart			
D. Must be prepared several times in advance before change is introduced			
E. Demands adult company constantly			
2. Attention			
A. Is easily distractible, shows fleeting attention			
B. Has difficulty paying attention, is difficult to reengage			
3. Sleep			
Wakes 3 or more times in the night and is unable to fall back to sleep			
4. Eating or Feeding			
A. Craves certain foods or drinks			
B. Is too distracted to stay seated for meals			
5. Dressing, Bathing, Touch			
A. Resists cuddling, pulls away or arches			
B. Hates sitting in car seat			
C. Resists being placed in certain positions, such as stomach or back			
6. Movement			
A. Is in constant movement—rocking, running about, unable to sit still for an activity			
B. Craves swinging and moving upside-down			
C. Is clumsy—falls, has poor balance, bumps into things			
7. Listening, Language and Sound			
A. Is distracted by sounds the average person doesn't notice			
B. Doesn't respond to verbal cues (hearing not a problem)			
C. Repeats or echoes previously heard words, phrases, or sentences			

continued

076-1643753-4

Infant/Toddler Symptom Checklist: 19 to 24 Months (continued)

	Never or Sometimes	Most Times	Past
8. Looking and Sight			
Becomes excited in crowded, bustling settings such as supermarkets, restaurants			
9. Attachment/Emotional Functioning			
A. Does not play with other children—withdraws or is aggressive			
B. Does not respond at all to limits, discipline			
C. Needs total control of the environment—"runs the show"			

How concerned are you about the symptoms checked above? (Circle one.)

Not concerned Slightly concerned Moderately concerned Very concerned

Comments:

Infant/Toddler Symptom Checklist:
19 to 24 Months

Name________________________________ Date______________

	Never or Sometimes	Most Times	Past
1. Self-Regulation			
A. Goes easily from whimper to intense cry			
B. Can't calm self effectively by sucking on pacifier, looking at toys, or listening to caregiver			
C. Is unable to wait for food or toy without falling apart			
D. Must be prepared several times in advance before change is introduced			
E. Demands adult company constantly			
2. Attention			
A. Is easily distractible, shows fleeting attention			
B. Has difficulty paying attention, is difficult to reengage			
3. Sleep			
Wakes 3 or more times in the night and is unable to fall back to sleep			
4. Eating or Feeding			
A. Craves certain foods or drinks			
B. Is too distracted to stay seated for meals			
5. Dressing, Bathing, Touch			
A. Resists cuddling, pulls away or arches			
B. Hates sitting in car seat			
C. Resists being placed in certain positions, such as stomach or back			
6. Movement			
A. Is in constant movement—rocking, running about, unable to sit still for an activity			
B. Craves swinging and moving upside-down			
C. Is clumsy—falls, has poor balance, bumps into things			
7. Listening, Language and Sound			
A. Is distracted by sounds the average person doesn't notice			
B. Doesn't respond to verbal cues (hearing not a problem)			
C. Repeats or echoes previously heard words, phrases, or sentences			

continued

076-1643753-4

Infant/Toddler Symptom Checklist:
19 to 24 Months (continued)

	Never or Sometimes	Most Times	Past
8. Looking and Sight			
Becomes excited in crowded, bustling settings such as supermarkets, restaurants			
9. Attachment/Emotional Functioning			
A. Does not play with other children—withdraws or is aggressive			
B. Does not respond at all to limits, discipline			
C. Needs total control of the environment—"runs the show"			

How concerned are you about the symptoms checked above? (Circle one.)

Not concerned   Slightly concerned   Moderately concerned   Very concerned

Comments:

Infant/Toddler Symptom Checklist:
19 to 24 Months

Name______________________________ Date______________

	Never or Sometimes	Most Times	Past
1. Self-Regulation			
A. Goes easily from whimper to intense cry			
B. Can't calm self effectively by sucking on pacifier, looking at toys, or listening to caregiver			
C. Is unable to wait for food or toy without falling apart			
D. Must be prepared several times in advance before change is introduced			
E. Demands adult company constantly			
2. Attention			
A. Is easily distractible, shows fleeting attention			
B. Has difficulty paying attention, is difficult to reengage			
3. Sleep			
Wakes 3 or more times in the night and is unable to fall back to sleep			
4. Eating or Feeding			
A. Craves certain foods or drinks			
B. Is too distracted to stay seated for meals			
5. Dressing, Bathing, Touch			
A. Resists cuddling, pulls away or arches			
B. Hates sitting in car seat			
C. Resists being placed in certain positions, such as stomach or back			
6. Movement			
A. Is in constant movement—rocking, running about, unable to sit still for an activity			
B. Craves swinging and moving upside-down			
C. Is clumsy—falls, has poor balance, bumps into things			
7. Listening, Language and Sound			
A. Is distracted by sounds the average person doesn't notice			
B. Doesn't respond to verbal cues (hearing not a problem)			
C. Repeats or echoes previously heard words, phrases, or sentences			

continued

076-1643753-4

Infant/Toddler Symptom Checklist: 19 to 24 Months (continued)

	Never or Sometimes	Most Times	Past
8. Looking and Sight			
Becomes excited in crowded, bustling settings such as supermarkets, restaurants			
9. Attachment/Emotional Functioning			
A. Does not play with other children—withdraws or is aggressive			
B. Does not respond at all to limits, discipline			
C. Needs total control of the environment—"runs the show"			

How concerned are you about the symptoms checked above? (Circle one.)

Not concerned   Slightly concerned   Moderately concerned   Very concerned

Comments:

Infant/Toddler Symptom Checklist:
19 to 24 Months

Name______________________________ Date______________

	Never or Sometimes	Most Times	Past
1. Self-Regulation			
A. Goes easily from whimper to intense cry			
B. Can't calm self effectively by sucking on pacifier, looking at toys, or listening to caregiver			
C. Is unable to wait for food or toy without falling apart			
D. Must be prepared several times in advance before change is introduced			
E. Demands adult company constantly			
2. Attention			
A. Is easily distractible, shows fleeting attention			
B. Has difficulty paying attention, is difficult to reengage			
3. Sleep			
Wakes 3 or more times in the night and is unable to fall back to sleep			
4. Eating or Feeding			
A. Craves certain foods or drinks			
B. Is too distracted to stay seated for meals			
5. Dressing, Bathing, Touch			
A. Resists cuddling, pulls away or arches			
B. Hates sitting in car seat			
C. Resists being placed in certain positions, such as stomach or back			
6. Movement			
A. Is in constant movement—rocking, running about, unable to sit still for an activity			
B. Craves swinging and moving upside-down			
C. Is clumsy—falls, has poor balance, bumps into things			
7. Listening, Language and Sound			
A. Is distracted by sounds the average person doesn't notice			
B. Doesn't respond to verbal cues (hearing not a problem)			
C. Repeats or echoes previously heard words, phrases, or sentences			

continued

076-1643753-4

Infant/Toddler Symptom Checklist: 19 to 24 Months (continued)

	Never or Sometimes	Most Times	Past
8. Looking and Sight			
Becomes excited in crowded, bustling settings such as supermarkets, restaurants			
9. Attachment/Emotional Functioning			
A. Does not play with other children—withdraws or is aggressive			
B. Does not respond at all to limits, discipline			
C. Needs total control of the environment—"runs the show"			

How concerned are you about the symptoms checked above? (Circle one.)

Not concerned Slightly concerned Moderately concerned Very concerned

Comments:

Infant/Toddler Symptom Checklist: 19 to 24 Months

Name__________________________________ Date________________

	Never or Sometimes	Most Times	Past
1. Self-Regulation			
A. Goes easily from whimper to intense cry			
B. Can't calm self effectively by sucking on pacifier, looking at toys, or listening to caregiver			
C. Is unable to wait for food or toy without falling apart			
D. Must be prepared several times in advance before change is introduced			
E. Demands adult company constantly			
2. Attention			
A. Is easily distractible, shows fleeting attention			
B. Has difficulty paying attention, is difficult to reengage			
3. Sleep			
Wakes 3 or more times in the night and is unable to fall back to sleep			
4. Eating or Feeding			
A. Craves certain foods or drinks			
B. Is too distracted to stay seated for meals			
5. Dressing, Bathing, Touch			
A. Resists cuddling, pulls away or arches			
B. Hates sitting in car seat			
C. Resists being placed in certain positions, such as stomach or back			
6. Movement			
A. Is in constant movement—rocking, running about, unable to sit still for an activity			
B. Craves swinging and moving upside-down			
C. Is clumsy—falls, has poor balance, bumps into things			
7. Listening, Language and Sound			
A. Is distracted by sounds the average person doesn't notice			
B. Doesn't respond to verbal cues (hearing not a problem)			
C. Repeats or echoes previously heard words, phrases, or sentences			

continued

076-1643753-4

Infant/Toddler Symptom Checklist:
19 to 24 Months (continued)

	Never or Sometimes	Most Times	Past
8. Looking and Sight			
Becomes excited in crowded, bustling settings such as supermarkets, restaurants			
9. Attachment/Emotional Functioning			
A. Does not play with other children—withdraws or is aggressive			
B. Does not respond at all to limits, discipline			
C. Needs total control of the environment—"runs the show"			

How concerned are you about the symptoms checked above? (Circle one.)

Not concerned Slightly concerned Moderately concerned Very concerned

Comments:

Infant/Toddler Symptom Checklist:
19 to 24 Months

Name____ Date______________

	Never or Sometimes	Most Times	Past
1. Self-Regulation			
A. Goes easily from whimper to intense cry			
B. Can't calm self effectively by sucking on pacifier, looking at toys, or listening to caregiver			
C. Is unable to wait for food or toy without falling apart			
D. Must be prepared several times in advance before change is introduced			
E. Demands adult company constantly			
2. Attention			
A. Is easily distractible, shows fleeting attention			
B. Has difficulty paying attention, is difficult to reengage			
3. Sleep			
Wakes 3 or more times in the night and is unable to fall back to sleep			
4. Eating or Feeding			
A. Craves certain foods or drinks			
B. Is too distracted to stay seated for meals			
5. Dressing, Bathing, Touch			
A. Resists cuddling, pulls away or arches			
B. Hates sitting in car seat			
C. Resists being placed in certain positions, such as stomach or back			
6. Movement			
A. Is in constant movement—rocking, running about, unable to sit still for an activity			
B. Craves swinging and moving upside-down			
C. Is clumsy—falls, has poor balance, bumps into things			
7. Listening, Language and Sound			
A. Is distracted by sounds the average person doesn't notice			
B. Doesn't respond to verbal cues (hearing not a problem)			
C. Repeats or echoes previously heard words, phrases, or sentences			

continued

076-1643753-4

Infant/Toddler Symptom Checklist:
19 to 24 Months (continued)

	Never or Sometimes	Most Times	Past
8. Looking and Sight			
Becomes excited in crowded, bustling settings such as supermarkets, restaurants			
9. Attachment/Emotional Functioning			
A. Does not play with other children—withdraws or is aggressive			
B. Does not respond at all to limits, discipline			
C. Needs total control of the environment—"runs the show"			

How concerned are you about the symptoms checked above? (Circle one.)

Not concerned   Slightly concerned   Moderately concerned   Very concerned

Comments:

Infant/Toddler Symptom Checklist:
19 to 24 Months

Name______________________________ Date______________

	Never or Sometimes	Most Times	Past
1. Self-Regulation			
A. Goes easily from whimper to intense cry			
B. Can't calm self effectively by sucking on pacifier, looking at toys, or listening to caregiver			
C. Is unable to wait for food or toy without falling apart			
D. Must be prepared several times in advance before change is introduced			
E. Demands adult company constantly			
2. Attention			
A. Is easily distractible, shows fleeting attention			
B. Has difficulty paying attention, is difficult to reengage			
3. Sleep			
Wakes 3 or more times in the night and is unable to fall back to sleep			
4. Eating or Feeding			
A. Craves certain foods or drinks			
B. Is too distracted to stay seated for meals			
5. Dressing, Bathing, Touch			
A. Resists cuddling, pulls away or arches			
B. Hates sitting in car seat			
C. Resists being placed in certain positions, such as stomach or back			
6. Movement			
A. Is in constant movement—rocking, running about, unable to sit still for an activity			
B. Craves swinging and moving upside-down			
C. Is clumsy—falls, has poor balance, bumps into things			
7. Listening, Language and Sound			
A. Is distracted by sounds the average person doesn't notice			
B. Doesn't respond to verbal cues (hearing not a problem)			
C. Repeats or echoes previously heard words, phrases, or sentences			

continued

076-1643753-4

Infant/Toddler Symptom Checklist:
19 to 24 Months (continued)

	Never or Sometimes	Most Times	Past
8. Looking and Sight			
Becomes excited in crowded, bustling settings such as supermarkets, restaurants			
9. Attachment/Emotional Functioning			
A. Does not play with other children—withdraws or is aggressive			
B. Does not respond at all to limits, discipline			
C. Needs total control of the environment—"runs the show"			

How concerned are you about the symptoms checked above? (Circle one.)

Not concerned   Slightly concerned   Moderately concerned   Very concerned

Comments:

Infant/Toddler Symptom Checklist:
19 to 24 Months

Name______________________ Date______________

	Never or Sometimes	Most Times	Past
1. Self-Regulation			
A. Goes easily from whimper to intense cry			
B. Can't calm self effectively by sucking on pacifier, looking at toys, or listening to caregiver			
C. Is unable to wait for food or toy without falling apart			
D. Must be prepared several times in advance before change is introduced			
E. Demands adult company constantly			
2. Attention			
A. Is easily distractible, shows fleeting attention			
B. Has difficulty paying attention, is difficult to reengage			
3. Sleep			
Wakes 3 or more times in the night and is unable to fall back to sleep			
4. Eating or Feeding			
A. Craves certain foods or drinks			
B. Is too distracted to stay seated for meals			
5. Dressing, Bathing, Touch			
A. Resists cuddling, pulls away or arches			
B. Hates sitting in car seat			
C. Resists being placed in certain positions, such as stomach or back			
6. Movement			
A. Is in constant movement—rocking, running about, unable to sit still for an activity			
B. Craves swinging and moving upside-down			
C. Is clumsy—falls, has poor balance, bumps into things			
7. Listening, Language and Sound			
A. Is distracted by sounds the average person doesn't notice			
B. Doesn't respond to verbal cues (hearing not a problem)			
C. Repeats or echoes previously heard words, phrases, or sentences			

continued

076-1643753-4

Infant/Toddler Symptom Checklist:
19 to 24 Months (continued)

	Never or Sometimes	Most Times	Past
8. Looking and Sight			
Becomes excited in crowded, bustling settings such as supermarkets, restaurants			
9. Attachment/Emotional Functioning			
A. Does not play with other children—withdraws or is aggressive			
B. Does not respond at all to limits, discipline			
C. Needs total control of the environment—"runs the show"			

How concerned are you about the symptoms checked above? (Circle one.)

Not concerned   Slightly concerned   Moderately concerned   Very concerned

Comments:

Infant/Toddler Symptom Checklist:
19 to 24 Months

Name______________________________ Date______________

	Never or Sometimes	Most Times	Past
1. Self-Regulation			
A. Goes easily from whimper to intense cry			
B. Can't calm self effectively by sucking on pacifier, looking at toys, or listening to caregiver			
C. Is unable to wait for food or toy without falling apart			
D. Must be prepared several times in advance before change is introduced			
E. Demands adult company constantly			
2. Attention			
A. Is easily distractible, shows fleeting attention			
B. Has difficulty paying attention, is difficult to reengage			
3. Sleep			
Wakes 3 or more times in the night and is unable to fall back to sleep			
4. Eating or Feeding			
A. Craves certain foods or drinks			
B. Is too distracted to stay seated for meals			
5. Dressing, Bathing, Touch			
A. Resists cuddling, pulls away or arches			
B. Hates sitting in car seat			
C. Resists being placed in certain positions, such as stomach or back			
6. Movement			
A. Is in constant movement—rocking, running about, unable to sit still for an activity			
B. Craves swinging and moving upside-down			
C. Is clumsy—falls, has poor balance, bumps into things			
7. Listening, Language and Sound			
A. Is distracted by sounds the average person doesn't notice			
B. Doesn't respond to verbal cues (hearing not a problem)			
C. Repeats or echoes previously heard words, phrases, or sentences			

continued

076-1643753-4

Infant/Toddler Symptom Checklist: 19 to 24 Months (continued)

	Never or Sometimes	Most Times	Past
8. Looking and Sight			
Becomes excited in crowded, bustling settings such as supermarkets, restaurants			
9. Attachment/Emotional Functioning			
A. Does not play with other children—withdraws or is aggressive			
B. Does not respond at all to limits, discipline			
C. Needs total control of the environment—"runs the show"			

How concerned are you about the symptoms checked above? (Circle one.)

Not concerned Slightly concerned Moderately concerned Very concerned

Comments:

Infant/Toddler Symptom Checklist:
19 to 24 Months

Name______________________________ Date______________

	Never or Sometimes	Most Times	Past
1. Self-Regulation			
A. Goes easily from whimper to intense cry			
B. Can't calm self effectively by sucking on pacifier, looking at toys, or listening to caregiver			
C. Is unable to wait for food or toy without falling apart			
D. Must be prepared several times in advance before change is introduced			
E. Demands adult company constantly			
2. Attention			
A. Is easily distractible, shows fleeting attention			
B. Has difficulty paying attention, is difficult to reengage			
3. Sleep			
Wakes 3 or more times in the night and is unable to fall back to sleep			
4. Eating or Feeding			
A. Craves certain foods or drinks			
B. Is too distracted to stay seated for meals			
5. Dressing, Bathing, Touch			
A. Resists cuddling, pulls away or arches			
B. Hates sitting in car seat			
C. Resists being placed in certain positions, such as stomach or back			
6. Movement			
A. Is in constant movement—rocking, running about, unable to sit still for an activity			
B. Craves swinging and moving upside-down			
C. Is clumsy—falls, has poor balance, bumps into things			
7. Listening, Language and Sound			
A. Is distracted by sounds the average person doesn't notice			
B. Doesn't respond to verbal cues (hearing not a problem)			
C. Repeats or echoes previously heard words, phrases, or sentences			

continued

076-1643753-4

Infant/Toddler Symptom Checklist: 19 to 24 Months (continued)

	Never or Sometimes	Most Times	Past
8. Looking and Sight			
Becomes excited in crowded, bustling settings such as supermarkets, restaurants			
9. Attachment/Emotional Functioning			
A. Does not play with other children—withdraws or is aggressive			
B. Does not respond at all to limits, discipline			
C. Needs total control of the environment—"runs the show"			

How concerned are you about the symptoms checked above? (Circle one.)

Not concerned   Slightly concerned   Moderately concerned   Very concerned

Comments:

Infant/Toddler Symptom Checklist:
25 to 30 Months

Name________________________________ Date______________

	Never or Sometimes	Most Times	Past
1. Self-Regulation			
A. Is frequently irritable, fussy			
B. Goes easily from whimper to intense cry			
C. Can't calm self effectively by sucking on pacifier, looking at toys, or listening to caregiver			
D. Is unable to wait for food or toy without falling apart			
E. Can't change from one activity to another without distress (Must be prepared several times in advance before change is introduced)			
F. Amount of time spent calming child during day (circle one): 15-30 minutes 1-2 hours 3 hours +			
2. Attention			
A. Is easily distractible, has fleeting attention			
B. Tunes out from activity, is difficult to reengage			
C. Can't shift focus easily from one object or activity to another			
3. Sleep			
Requires extensive help to fall asleep; *specify:* rocking, long walks, stroking hair, car ride, other: ______________			
4. Dressing, Bathing, Touch			
Is distressed when face or hair washed			
5. Movement			
A. Is in constant movement, rocking, running about, unable to sit still for an activity			
B. Is fearful of being swung in air, swings, merry-go-rounds			
6. Looking and Sight			
A. Is sensitive to bright lights—cries or closes eyes			
B. Becomes excited in crowded, bustling settings such as supermarkets, restaurants			
7. Attachment/Emotional Functioning			
A. Appears anxious or fearful of new people, situations			
B. Needs total control of the environment—"runs the show"			

continued

076-1643753-5

Infant/Toddler Symptom Checklist:
25 to 30 Months (continued)

How concerned are you about the symptoms checked above? (Circle one.)

Not concerned Slightly concerned Moderately concerned Very concerned

---

Comments:

Infant/Toddler Symptom Checklist: 25 to 30 Months

Name______________________ Date____________

	Never or Sometimes	Most Times	Past
1. Self-Regulation			
A. Is frequently irritable, fussy			
B. Goes easily from whimper to intense cry			
C. Can't calm self effectively by sucking on pacifier, looking at toys, or listening to caregiver			
D. Is unable to wait for food or toy without falling apart			
E. Can't change from one activity to another without distress (Must be prepared several times in advance before change is introduced)			
F. Amount of time spent calming child during day (circle one): 15-30 minutes 1-2 hours 3 hours +			
2. Attention			
A. Is easily distractible, has fleeting attention			
B. Tunes out from activity, is difficult to reengage			
C. Can't shift focus easily from one object or activity to another			
3. Sleep			
Requires extensive help to fall asleep; *specify:* rocking, long walks, stroking hair, car ride, other: ______________			
4. Dressing, Bathing, Touch			
Is distressed when face or hair washed			
5. Movement			
A. Is in constant movement, rocking, running about, unable to sit still for an activity			
B. Is fearful of being swung in air, swings, merry-go-rounds			
6. Looking and Sight			
A. Is sensitive to bright lights—cries or closes eyes			
B. Becomes excited in crowded, bustling settings such as supermarkets, restaurants			
7. Attachment/Emotional Functioning			
A. Appears anxious or fearful of new people, situations			
B. Needs total control of the environment—"runs the show"			

continued

076-1643753-5

Infant/Toddler Symptom Checklist:
25 to 30 Months (continued)

How concerned are you about the symptoms checked above? (Circle one.)

Not concerned   Slightly concerned   Moderately concerned   Very concerned

---

Comments:

Infant/Toddler Symptom Checklist:
25 to 30 Months

Name________________________________ Date______________

	Never or Sometimes	Most Times	Past
1. Self-Regulation			
A. Is frequently irritable, fussy			
B. Goes easily from whimper to intense cry			
C. Can't calm self effectively by sucking on pacifier, looking at toys, or listening to caregiver			
D. Is unable to wait for food or toy without falling apart			
E. Can't change from one activity to another without distress (Must be prepared several times in advance before change is introduced)			
F. Amount of time spent calming child during day (circle one): 15-30 minutes 1-2 hours 3 hours +			
2. Attention			
A. Is easily distractible, has fleeting attention			
B. Tunes out from activity, is difficult to reengage			
C. Can't shift focus easily from one object or activity to another			
3. Sleep			
Requires extensive help to fall asleep; *specify:* rocking, long walks, stroking hair, car ride, other: ______________			
4. Dressing, Bathing, Touch			
Is distressed when face or hair washed			
5. Movement			
A. Is in constant movement, rocking, running about, unable to sit still for an activity			
B. Is fearful of being swung in air, swings, merry-go-rounds			
6. Looking and Sight			
A. Is sensitive to bright lights—cries or closes eyes			
B. Becomes excited in crowded, bustling settings such as supermarkets, restaurants			
7. Attachment/Emotional Functioning			
A. Appears anxious or fearful of new people, situations			
B. Needs total control of the environment—"runs the show"			

continued

076-1643753-5

Infant/Toddler Symptom Checklist:
25 to 30 Months (continued)

How concerned are you about the symptoms checked above? (Circle one.)

Not concerned   Slightly concerned   Moderately concerned   Very concerned

---

Comments:

Infant/Toddler Symptom Checklist:
25 to 30 Months

Name_______________________________ Date_______________

	Never or Sometimes	Most Times	Past
1. Self-Regulation			
A. Is frequently irritable, fussy			
B. Goes easily from whimper to intense cry			
C. Can't calm self effectively by sucking on pacifier, looking at toys, or listening to caregiver			
D. Is unable to wait for food or toy without falling apart			
E. Can't change from one activity to another without distress (Must be prepared several times in advance before change is introduced)			
F. Amount of time spent calming child during day (circle one): 15-30 minutes 1-2 hours 3 hours +			
2. Attention			
A. Is easily distractible, has fleeting attention			
B. Tunes out from activity, is difficult to reengage			
C. Can't shift focus easily from one object or activity to another			
3. Sleep			
Requires extensive help to fall asleep; *specify:* rocking, long walks, stroking hair, car ride, other: ____________________			
4. Dressing, Bathing, Touch			
Is distressed when face or hair washed			
5. Movement			
A. Is in constant movement, rocking, running about, unable to sit still for an activity			
B. Is fearful of being swung in air, swings, merry-go-rounds			
6. Looking and Sight			
A. Is sensitive to bright lights—cries or closes eyes			
B. Becomes excited in crowded, bustling settings such as supermarkets, restaurants			
7. Attachment/Emotional Functioning			
A. Appears anxious or fearful of new people, situations			
B. Needs total control of the environment—"runs the show"			

continued

076-1643753-5

Infant/Toddler Symptom Checklist:
25 to 30 Months (continued)

How concerned are you about the symptoms checked above? (Circle one.)

Not concerned   Slightly concerned   Moderately concerned   Very concerned

Comments:

Infant/Toddler Symptom Checklist:
25 to 30 Months

Name________________________________ Date______________

	Never or Sometimes	Most Times	Past
1. Self-Regulation			
A. Is frequently irritable, fussy			
B. Goes easily from whimper to intense cry			
C. Can't calm self effectively by sucking on pacifier, looking at toys, or listening to caregiver			
D. Is unable to wait for food or toy without falling apart			
E. Can't change from one activity to another without distress (Must be prepared several times in advance before change is introduced)			
F. Amount of time spent calming child during day (circle one): 15-30 minutes 1-2 hours 3 hours +			
2. Attention			
A. Is easily distractible, has fleeting attention			
B. Tunes out from activity, is difficult to reengage			
C. Can't shift focus easily from one object or activity to another			
3. Sleep			
Requires extensive help to fall asleep; *specify:* rocking, long walks, stroking hair, car ride, other: ____________			
4. Dressing, Bathing, Touch			
Is distressed when face or hair washed			
5. Movement			
A. Is in constant movement, rocking, running about, unable to sit still for an activity			
B. Is fearful of being swung in air, swings, merry-go-rounds			
6. Looking and Sight			
A. Is sensitive to bright lights—cries or closes eyes			
B. Becomes excited in crowded, bustling settings such as supermarkets, restaurants			
7. Attachment/Emotional Functioning			
A. Appears anxious or fearful of new people, situations			
B. Needs total control of the environment—"runs the show"			

continued

076-1643753-5

Infant/Toddler Symptom Checklist:
25 to 30 Months (continued)

How concerned are you about the symptoms checked above? (Circle one.)

Not concerned Slightly concerned Moderately concerned Very concerned

Comments:

Infant/Toddler Symptom Checklist:
25 to 30 Months

Name_______________________________ Date______________

	Never or Sometimes	Most Times	Past
1. Self-Regulation			
A. Is frequently irritable, fussy			
B. Goes easily from whimper to intense cry			
C. Can't calm self effectively by sucking on pacifier, looking at toys, or listening to caregiver			
D. Is unable to wait for food or toy without falling apart			
E. Can't change from one activity to another without distress (Must be prepared several times in advance before change is introduced)			

F. Amount of time spent calming child during day (circle one):

15-30 minutes   1-2 hours   3 hours +

	Never or Sometimes	Most Times	Past
2. Attention			
A. Is easily distractible, has fleeting attention			
B. Tunes out from activity, is difficult to reengage			
C. Can't shift focus easily from one object or activity to another			
3. Sleep			
Requires extensive help to fall asleep; *specify:* rocking, long walks, stroking hair, car ride, other: ______________________			
4. Dressing, Bathing, Touch			
Is distressed when face or hair washed			
5. Movement			
A. Is in constant movement, rocking, running about, unable to sit still for an activity			
B. Is fearful of being swung in air, swings, merry-go-rounds			
6. Looking and Sight			
A. Is sensitive to bright lights—cries or closes eyes			
B. Becomes excited in crowded, bustling settings such as supermarkets, restaurants			
7. Attachment/Emotional Functioning			
A. Appears anxious or fearful of new people, situations			
B. Needs total control of the environment—"runs the show"			

continued

Infant/Toddler Symptom Checklist:
25 to 30 Months (continued)

How concerned are you about the symptoms checked above? (Circle one.)

Not concerned   Slightly concerned   Moderately concerned   Very concerned

Comments:

Infant/Toddler Symptom Checklist:
25 to 30 Months

Name________________________ Date______________

	Never or Sometimes	Most Times	Past
1. Self-Regulation			
A. Is frequently irritable, fussy			
B. Goes easily from whimper to intense cry			
C. Can't calm self effectively by sucking on pacifier, looking at toys, or listening to caregiver			
D. Is unable to wait for food or toy without falling apart			
E. Can't change from one activity to another without distress (Must be prepared several times in advance before change is introduced)			
F. Amount of time spent calming child during day (circle one): 15-30 minutes 1-2 hours 3 hours +			
2. Attention			
A. Is easily distractible, has fleeting attention			
B. Tunes out from activity, is difficult to reengage			
C. Can't shift focus easily from one object or activity to another			
3. Sleep			
Requires extensive help to fall asleep; *specify:* rocking, long walks, stroking hair, car ride, other: ______________			
4. Dressing, Bathing, Touch			
Is distressed when face or hair washed			
5. Movement			
A. Is in constant movement, rocking, running about, unable to sit still for an activity			
B. Is fearful of being swung in air, swings, merry-go-rounds			
6. Looking and Sight			
A. Is sensitive to bright lights—cries or closes eyes			
B. Becomes excited in crowded, bustling settings such as supermarkets, restaurants			
7. Attachment/Emotional Functioning			
A. Appears anxious or fearful of new people, situations			
B. Needs total control of the environment—"runs the show"			

continued

Infant/Toddler Symptom Checklist:
25 to 30 Months (continued)

How concerned are you about the symptoms checked above? (Circle one.)

Not concerned   Slightly concerned   Moderately concerned   Very concerned

---

Comments:

Infant/Toddler Symptom Checklist:
25 to 30 Months

Name______________________________ Date______________

	Never or Sometimes	Most Times	Past
1. Self-Regulation			
A. Is frequently irritable, fussy			
B. Goes easily from whimper to intense cry			
C. Can't calm self effectively by sucking on pacifier, looking at toys, or listening to caregiver			
D. Is unable to wait for food or toy without falling apart			
E. Can't change from one activity to another without distress (Must be prepared several times in advance before change is introduced)			
F. Amount of time spent calming child during day (circle one): 15-30 minutes 1-2 hours 3 hours +			
2. Attention			
A. Is easily distractible, has fleeting attention			
B. Tunes out from activity, is difficult to reengage			
C. Can't shift focus easily from one object or activity to another			
3. Sleep			
Requires extensive help to fall asleep; *specify:* rocking, long walks, stroking hair, car ride, other: ______________			
4. Dressing, Bathing, Touch			
Is distressed when face or hair washed			
5. Movement			
A. Is in constant movement, rocking, running about, unable to sit still for an activity			
B. Is fearful of being swung in air, swings, merry-go-rounds			
6. Looking and Sight			
A. Is sensitive to bright lights—cries or closes eyes			
B. Becomes excited in crowded, bustling settings such as supermarkets, restaurants			
7. Attachment/Emotional Functioning			
A. Appears anxious or fearful of new people, situations			
B. Needs total control of the environment—"runs the show"			

continued

076-1643753-5

Infant/Toddler Symptom Checklist:
25 to 30 Months (continued)

How concerned are you about the symptoms checked above? (Circle one.)

Not concerned Slightly concerned Moderately concerned Very concerned

---

Comments:

Infant/Toddler Symptom Checklist:
25 to 30 Months

Name________________________ Date______________

	Never or Sometimes	Most Times	Past
1. Self-Regulation			
A. Is frequently irritable, fussy			
B. Goes easily from whimper to intense cry			
C. Can't calm self effectively by sucking on pacifier, looking at toys, or listening to caregiver			
D. Is unable to wait for food or toy without falling apart			
E. Can't change from one activity to another without distress (Must be prepared several times in advance before change is introduced)			
F. Amount of time spent calming child during day (circle one): 15-30 minutes 1-2 hours 3 hours +			
2. Attention			
A. Is easily distractible, has fleeting attention			
B. Tunes out from activity, is difficult to reengage			
C. Can't shift focus easily from one object or activity to another			
3. Sleep			
Requires extensive help to fall asleep; *specify:* rocking, long walks, stroking hair, car ride, other: ______________			
4. Dressing, Bathing, Touch			
Is distressed when face or hair washed			
5. Movement			
A. Is in constant movement, rocking, running about, unable to sit still for an activity			
B. Is fearful of being swung in air, swings, merry-go-rounds			
6. Looking and Sight			
A. Is sensitive to bright lights—cries or closes eyes			
B. Becomes excited in crowded, bustling settings such as supermarkets, restaurants			
7. Attachment/Emotional Functioning			
A. Appears anxious or fearful of new people, situations			
B. Needs total control of the environment—"runs the show"			

continued

076-1643753-5

Infant/Toddler Symptom Checklist: 25 to 30 Months (continued)

How concerned are you about the symptoms checked above? (Circle one.)

Not concerned   Slightly concerned   Moderately concerned   Very concerned

Comments:

Infant/Toddler Symptom Checklist:
25 to 30 Months

Name____ Date______________

	Never or Sometimes	Most Times	Past
1. Self-Regulation			
A. Is frequently irritable, fussy			
B. Goes easily from whimper to intense cry			
C. Can't calm self effectively by sucking on pacifier, looking at toys, or listening to caregiver			
D. Is unable to wait for food or toy without falling apart			
E. Can't change from one activity to another without distress (Must be prepared several times in advance before change is introduced)			
F. Amount of time spent calming child during day (circle one): 15-30 minutes 1-2 hours 3 hours +			
2. Attention			
A. Is easily distractible, has fleeting attention			
B. Tunes out from activity, is difficult to reengage			
C. Can't shift focus easily from one object or activity to another			
3. Sleep			
Requires extensive help to fall asleep; *specify:* rocking, long walks, stroking hair, car ride, other: ______________________________			
4. Dressing, Bathing, Touch			
Is distressed when face or hair washed			
5. Movement			
A. Is in constant movement, rocking, running about, unable to sit still for an activity			
B. Is fearful of being swung in air, swings, merry-go-rounds			
6. Looking and Sight			
A. Is sensitive to bright lights—cries or closes eyes			
B. Becomes excited in crowded, bustling settings such as supermarkets, restaurants			
7. Attachment/Emotional Functioning			
A. Appears anxious or fearful of new people, situations			
B. Needs total control of the environment—"runs the show"			

continued

076-1643753-5

Infant/Toddler Symptom Checklist:
25 to 30 Months (continued)

How concerned are you about the symptoms checked above? (Circle one.)

Not concerned   Slightly concerned   Moderately concerned   Very concerned

Comments:

Infant/Toddler Symptom Checklist:
25 to 30 Months

Name________________________________ Date______________

	Never or Sometimes	Most Times	Past
1. Self-Regulation			
A. Is frequently irritable, fussy			
B. Goes easily from whimper to intense cry			
C. Can't calm self effectively by sucking on pacifier, looking at toys, or listening to caregiver			
D. Is unable to wait for food or toy without falling apart			
E. Can't change from one activity to another without distress (Must be prepared several times in advance before change is introduced)			
F. Amount of time spent calming child during day (circle one): 15-30 minutes 1-2 hours 3 hours +			
2. Attention			
A. Is easily distractible, has fleeting attention			
B. Tunes out from activity, is difficult to reengage			
C. Can't shift focus easily from one object or activity to another			
3. Sleep			
Requires extensive help to fall asleep; *specify:* rocking, long walks, stroking hair, car ride, other: ______________			
4. Dressing, Bathing, Touch			
Is distressed when face or hair washed			
5. Movement			
A. Is in constant movement, rocking, running about, unable to sit still for an activity			
B. Is fearful of being swung in air, swings, merry-go-rounds			
6. Looking and Sight			
A. Is sensitive to bright lights—cries or closes eyes			
B. Becomes excited in crowded, bustling settings such as supermarkets, restaurants			
7. Attachment/Emotional Functioning			
A. Appears anxious or fearful of new people, situations			
B. Needs total control of the environment—"runs the show"			

continued

076-1643753-5

Infant/Toddler Symptom Checklist:
25 to 30 Months (continued)

How concerned are you about the symptoms checked above? (Circle one.)

Not concerned Slightly concerned Moderately concerned Very concerned

Comments:

Infant/Toddler Symptom Checklist:
25 to 30 Months

Name________________________________ Date______________

	Never or Sometimes	Most Times	Past
1. Self-Regulation			
A. Is frequently irritable, fussy			
B. Goes easily from whimper to intense cry			
C. Can't calm self effectively by sucking on pacifier, looking at toys, or listening to caregiver			
D. Is unable to wait for food or toy without falling apart			
E. Can't change from one activity to another without distress (Must be prepared several times in advance before change is introduced)			
F. Amount of time spent calming child during day (circle one): 15-30 minutes 1-2 hours 3 hours +			
2. Attention			
A. Is easily distractible, has fleeting attention			
B. Tunes out from activity, is difficult to reengage			
C. Can't shift focus easily from one object or activity to another			
3. Sleep			
Requires extensive help to fall asleep; *specify:* rocking, long walks, stroking hair, car ride, other: ______________			
4. Dressing, Bathing, Touch			
Is distressed when face or hair washed			
5. Movement			
A. Is in constant movement, rocking, running about, unable to sit still for an activity			
B. Is fearful of being swung in air, swings, merry-go-rounds			
6. Looking and Sight			
A. Is sensitive to bright lights—cries or closes eyes			
B. Becomes excited in crowded, bustling settings such as supermarkets, restaurants			
7. Attachment/Emotional Functioning			
A. Appears anxious or fearful of new people, situations			
B. Needs total control of the environment—"runs the show"			

continued

076-1643753-5

Infant/Toddler Symptom Checklist:
25 to 30 Months (continued)

How concerned are you about the symptoms checked above? (Circle one.)

Not concerned   Slightly concerned   Moderately concerned   Very concerned

---

Comments:

Infant/Toddler Symptom Checklist:
25 to 30 Months

Name________________________________ Date______________

	Never or Sometimes	Most Times	Past
1. Self-Regulation			
A. Is frequently irritable, fussy			
B. Goes easily from whimper to intense cry			
C. Can't calm self effectively by sucking on pacifier, looking at toys, or listening to caregiver			
D. Is unable to wait for food or toy without falling apart			
E. Can't change from one activity to another without distress (Must be prepared several times in advance before change is introduced)			
F. Amount of time spent calming child during day (circle one): 15-30 minutes 1-2 hours 3 hours +			
2. Attention			
A. Is easily distractible, has fleeting attention			
B. Tunes out from activity, is difficult to reengage			
C. Can't shift focus easily from one object or activity to another			
3. Sleep			
Requires extensive help to fall asleep; *specify:* rocking, long walks, stroking hair, car ride, other: ______________________			
4. Dressing, Bathing, Touch			
Is distressed when face or hair washed			
5. Movement			
A. Is in constant movement, rocking, running about, unable to sit still for an activity			
B. Is fearful of being swung in air, swings, merry-go-rounds			
6. Looking and Sight			
A. Is sensitive to bright lights—cries or closes eyes			
B. Becomes excited in crowded, bustling settings such as supermarkets, restaurants			
7. Attachment/Emotional Functioning			
A. Appears anxious or fearful of new people, situations			
B. Needs total control of the environment—"runs the show"			

continued

076-1643753-5

Infant/Toddler Symptom Checklist:
25 to 30 Months (continued)

How concerned are you about the symptoms checked above? (Circle one.)

Not concerned   Slightly concerned   Moderately concerned   Very concerned

---

Comments:

Infant/Toddler Symptom Checklist:
25 to 30 Months

Name______________________ Date__________

	Never or Sometimes	Most Times	Past
1. Self-Regulation			
A. Is frequently irritable, fussy			
B. Goes easily from whimper to intense cry			
C. Can't calm self effectively by sucking on pacifier, looking at toys, or listening to caregiver			
D. Is unable to wait for food or toy without falling apart			
E. Can't change from one activity to another without distress (Must be prepared several times in advance before change is introduced)			
F. Amount of time spent calming child during day (circle one): 15-30 minutes 1-2 hours 3 hours +			
2. Attention			
A. Is easily distractible, has fleeting attention			
B. Tunes out from activity, is difficult to reengage			
C. Can't shift focus easily from one object or activity to another			
3. Sleep			
Requires extensive help to fall asleep; *specify:* rocking, long walks, stroking hair, car ride, other: ____________			
4. Dressing, Bathing, Touch			
Is distressed when face or hair washed			
5. Movement			
A. Is in constant movement, rocking, running about, unable to sit still for an activity			
B. Is fearful of being swung in air, swings, merry-go-rounds			
6. Looking and Sight			
A. Is sensitive to bright lights—cries or closes eyes			
B. Becomes excited in crowded, bustling settings such as supermarkets, restaurants			
7. Attachment/Emotional Functioning			
A. Appears anxious or fearful of new people, situations			
B. Needs total control of the environment—"runs the show"			

continued

076-1643753-5

Infant/Toddler Symptom Checklist:
25 to 30 Months (continued)

How concerned are you about the symptoms checked above? (Circle one.)

Not concerned   Slightly concerned   Moderately concerned   Very concerned

Comments:

Infant/Toddler Symptom Checklist:
25 to 30 Months

Name____ Date________________

	Never or Sometimes	Most Times	Past
1. Self-Regulation			
A. Is frequently irritable, fussy			
B. Goes easily from whimper to intense cry			
C. Can't calm self effectively by sucking on pacifier, looking at toys, or listening to caregiver			
D. Is unable to wait for food or toy without falling apart			
E. Can't change from one activity to another without distress (Must be prepared several times in advance before change is introduced)			
F. Amount of time spent calming child during day (circle one): 15-30 minutes 1-2 hours 3 hours +			
2. Attention			
A. Is easily distractible, has fleeting attention			
B. Tunes out from activity, is difficult to reengage			
C. Can't shift focus easily from one object or activity to another			
3. Sleep			
Requires extensive help to fall asleep; *specify:* rocking, long walks, stroking hair, car ride, other: ______________________			
4. Dressing, Bathing, Touch			
Is distressed when face or hair washed			
5. Movement			
A. Is in constant movement, rocking, running about, unable to sit still for an activity			
B. Is fearful of being swung in air, swings, merry-go-rounds			
6. Looking and Sight			
A. Is sensitive to bright lights—cries or closes eyes			
B. Becomes excited in crowded, bustling settings such as supermarkets, restaurants			
7. Attachment/Emotional Functioning			
A. Appears anxious or fearful of new people, situations			
B. Needs total control of the environment—"runs the show"			

continued

Infant/Toddler Symptom Checklist:
25 to 30 Months (continued)

How concerned are you about the symptoms checked above? (Circle one.)

Not concerned Slightly concerned Moderately concerned Very concerned

---

Comments:

Infant/Toddler Symptom Checklist: 25 to 30 Months

Name________________________________ Date______________

	Never or Sometimes	Most Times	Past
1. Self-Regulation			
A. Is frequently irritable, fussy			
B. Goes easily from whimper to intense cry			
C. Can't calm self effectively by sucking on pacifier, looking at toys, or listening to caregiver			
D. Is unable to wait for food or toy without falling apart			
E. Can't change from one activity to another without distress (Must be prepared several times in advance before change is introduced)			
F. Amount of time spent calming child during day (circle one): 15-30 minutes 1-2 hours 3 hours +			
2. Attention			
A. Is easily distractible, has fleeting attention			
B. Tunes out from activity, is difficult to reengage			
C. Can't shift focus easily from one object or activity to another			
3. Sleep			
Requires extensive help to fall asleep; *specify:* rocking, long walks, stroking hair, car ride, other: ______________			
4. Dressing, Bathing, Touch			
Is distressed when face or hair washed			
5. Movement			
A. Is in constant movement, rocking, running about, unable to sit still for an activity			
B. Is fearful of being swung in air, swings, merry-go-rounds			
6. Looking and Sight			
A. Is sensitive to bright lights—cries or closes eyes			
B. Becomes excited in crowded, bustling settings such as supermarkets, restaurants			
7. Attachment/Emotional Functioning			
A. Appears anxious or fearful of new people, situations			
B. Needs total control of the environment—"runs the show"			

continued

076-1643753-5

Infant/Toddler Symptom Checklist:
25 to 30 Months (continued)

How concerned are you about the symptoms checked above? (Circle one.)

Not concerned Slightly concerned Moderately concerned Very concerned

---

Comments:

Infant/Toddler Symptom Checklist:
25 to 30 Months

Name_______________________ Date___________

	Never or Sometimes	Most Times	Past
1. Self-Regulation			
A. Is frequently irritable, fussy			
B. Goes easily from whimper to intense cry			
C. Can't calm self effectively by sucking on pacifier, looking at toys, or listening to caregiver			
D. Is unable to wait for food or toy without falling apart			
E. Can't change from one activity to another without distress (Must be prepared several times in advance before change is introduced)			
F. Amount of time spent calming child during day (circle one): 15-30 minutes 1-2 hours 3 hours +			
2. Attention			
A. Is easily distractible, has fleeting attention			
B. Tunes out from activity, is difficult to reengage			
C. Can't shift focus easily from one object or activity to another			
3. Sleep			
Requires extensive help to fall asleep; *specify:* rocking, long walks, stroking hair, car ride, other: ______________			
4. Dressing, Bathing, Touch			
Is distressed when face or hair washed			
5. Movement			
A. Is in constant movement, rocking, running about, unable to sit still for an activity			
B. Is fearful of being swung in air, swings, merry-go-rounds			
6. Looking and Sight			
A. Is sensitive to bright lights—cries or closes eyes			
B. Becomes excited in crowded, bustling settings such as supermarkets, restaurants			
7. Attachment/Emotional Functioning			
A. Appears anxious or fearful of new people, situations			
B. Needs total control of the environment—"runs the show"			

continued

076-1643753-5

Infant/Toddler Symptom Checklist:
25 to 30 Months (continued)

How concerned are you about the symptoms checked above? (Circle one.)

Not concerned   Slightly concerned   Moderately concerned   Very concerned

Comments:

Infant/Toddler Symptom Checklist: 25 to 30 Months

Name_______________________________________ Date_______________

	Never or Sometimes	Most Times	Past
1. Self-Regulation			
A. Is frequently irritable, fussy			
B. Goes easily from whimper to intense cry			
C. Can't calm self effectively by sucking on pacifier, looking at toys, or listening to caregiver			
D. Is unable to wait for food or toy without falling apart			
E. Can't change from one activity to another without distress (Must be prepared several times in advance before change is introduced)			
F. Amount of time spent calming child during day (circle one): 15-30 minutes 1-2 hours 3 hours +			
2. Attention			
A. Is easily distractible, has fleeting attention			
B. Tunes out from activity, is difficult to reengage			
C. Can't shift focus easily from one object or activity to another			
3. Sleep			
Requires extensive help to fall asleep; *specify:* rocking, long walks, stroking hair, car ride, other: ______________________			
4. Dressing, Bathing, Touch			
Is distressed when face or hair washed			
5. Movement			
A. Is in constant movement, rocking, running about, unable to sit still for an activity			
B. Is fearful of being swung in air, swings, merry-go-rounds			
6. Looking and Sight			
A. Is sensitive to bright lights—cries or closes eyes			
B. Becomes excited in crowded, bustling settings such as supermarkets, restaurants			
7. Attachment/Emotional Functioning			
A. Appears anxious or fearful of new people, situations			
B. Needs total control of the environment—"runs the show"			

continued

076-1643753-5

Infant/Toddler Symptom Checklist:
25 to 30 Months (continued)

How concerned are you about the symptoms checked above? (Circle one.)

Not concerned   Slightly concerned   Moderately concerned   Very concerned

Comments:

Infant/Toddler Symptom Checklist: 25 to 30 Months

Name______________________________________ Date______________

	Never or Sometimes	Most Times	Past
1. Self-Regulation			
A. Is frequently irritable, fussy			
B. Goes easily from whimper to intense cry			
C. Can't calm self effectively by sucking on pacifier, looking at toys, or listening to caregiver			
D. Is unable to wait for food or toy without falling apart			
E. Can't change from one activity to another without distress (Must be prepared several times in advance before change is introduced)			
F. Amount of time spent calming child during day (circle one): 15-30 minutes 1-2 hours 3 hours +			
2. Attention			
A. Is easily distractible, has fleeting attention			
B. Tunes out from activity, is difficult to reengage			
C. Can't shift focus easily from one object or activity to another			
3. Sleep			
Requires extensive help to fall asleep; *specify:* rocking, long walks, stroking hair, car ride, other: ______________________			
4. Dressing, Bathing, Touch			
Is distressed when face or hair washed			
5. Movement			
A. Is in constant movement, rocking, running about, unable to sit still for an activity			
B. Is fearful of being swung in air, swings, merry-go-rounds			
6. Looking and Sight			
A. Is sensitive to bright lights—cries or closes eyes			
B. Becomes excited in crowded, bustling settings such as supermarkets, restaurants			
7. Attachment/Emotional Functioning			
A. Appears anxious or fearful of new people, situations			
B. Needs total control of the environment—"runs the show"			

continued

076-1643753-5

Infant/Toddler Symptom Checklist:
25 to 30 Months (continued)

How concerned are you about the symptoms checked above? (Circle one.)

Not concerned   Slightly concerned   Moderately concerned   Very concerned

Comments:

Infant/Toddler Symptom Checklist:
25 to 30 Months

Name______________________________ Date______________

	Never or Sometimes	Most Times	Past
1. Self-Regulation			
A. Is frequently irritable, fussy			
B. Goes easily from whimper to intense cry			
C. Can't calm self effectively by sucking on pacifier, looking at toys, or listening to caregiver			
D. Is unable to wait for food or toy without falling apart			
E. Can't change from one activity to another without distress (Must be prepared several times in advance before change is introduced)			
F. Amount of time spent calming child during day (circle one): 15-30 minutes 1-2 hours 3 hours +			
2. Attention			
A. Is easily distractible, has fleeting attention			
B. Tunes out from activity, is difficult to reengage			
C. Can't shift focus easily from one object or activity to another			
3. Sleep			
Requires extensive help to fall asleep; *specify:* rocking, long walks, stroking hair, car ride, other: ______________			
4. Dressing, Bathing, Touch			
Is distressed when face or hair washed			
5. Movement			
A. Is in constant movement, rocking, running about, unable to sit still for an activity			
B. Is fearful of being swung in air, swings, merry-go-rounds			
6. Looking and Sight			
A. Is sensitive to bright lights—cries or closes eyes			
B. Becomes excited in crowded, bustling settings such as supermarkets, restaurants			
7. Attachment/Emotional Functioning			
A. Appears anxious or fearful of new people, situations			
B. Needs total control of the environment—"runs the show"			

continued

076-1643753-5

Infant/Toddler Symptom Checklist:
25 to 30 Months (continued)

How concerned are you about the symptoms checked above? (Circle one.)

Not concerned   Slightly concerned   Moderately concerned   Very concerned

Comments:

Infant/Toddler Symptom Checklist: 25 to 30 Months

Name______________________________ Date______________

	Never or Sometimes	Most Times	Past
1. Self-Regulation			
A. Is frequently irritable, fussy			
B. Goes easily from whimper to intense cry			
C. Can't calm self effectively by sucking on pacifier, looking at toys, or listening to caregiver			
D. Is unable to wait for food or toy without falling apart			
E. Can't change from one activity to another without distress (Must be prepared several times in advance before change is introduced)			
F. Amount of time spent calming child during day (circle one): 15-30 minutes 1-2 hours 3 hours +			
2. Attention			
A. Is easily distractible, has fleeting attention			
B. Tunes out from activity, is difficult to reengage			
C. Can't shift focus easily from one object or activity to another			
3. Sleep			
Requires extensive help to fall asleep; *specify:* rocking, long walks, stroking hair, car ride, other: ______________			
4. Dressing, Bathing, Touch			
Is distressed when face or hair washed			
5. Movement			
A. Is in constant movement, rocking, running about, unable to sit still for an activity			
B. Is fearful of being swung in air, swings, merry-go-rounds			
6. Looking and Sight			
A. Is sensitive to bright lights—cries or closes eyes			
B. Becomes excited in crowded, bustling settings such as supermarkets, restaurants			
7. Attachment/Emotional Functioning			
A. Appears anxious or fearful of new people, situations			
B. Needs total control of the environment—"runs the show"			

continued

076-1643753-5

Infant/Toddler Symptom Checklist:
25 to 30 Months (continued)

How concerned are you about the symptoms checked above? (Circle one.)

Not concerned   Slightly concerned   Moderately concerned   Very concerned

---

Comments:

Infant/Toddler Symptom Checklist: 25 to 30 Months

Name________________________________ Date______________

	Never or Sometimes	Most Times	Past
1. Self-Regulation			
A. Is frequently irritable, fussy			
B. Goes easily from whimper to intense cry			
C. Can't calm self effectively by sucking on pacifier, looking at toys, or listening to caregiver			
D. Is unable to wait for food or toy without falling apart			
E. Can't change from one activity to another without distress (Must be prepared several times in advance before change is introduced)			
F. Amount of time spent calming child during day (circle one): 15-30 minutes 1-2 hours 3 hours +			
2. Attention			
A. Is easily distractible, has fleeting attention			
B. Tunes out from activity, is difficult to reengage			
C. Can't shift focus easily from one object or activity to another			
3. Sleep			
Requires extensive help to fall asleep; *specify:* rocking, long walks, stroking hair, car ride, other: ____________			
4. Dressing, Bathing, Touch			
Is distressed when face or hair washed			
5. Movement			
A. Is in constant movement, rocking, running about, unable to sit still for an activity			
B. Is fearful of being swung in air, swings, merry-go-rounds			
6. Looking and Sight			
A. Is sensitive to bright lights—cries or closes eyes			
B. Becomes excited in crowded, bustling settings such as supermarkets, restaurants			
7. Attachment/Emotional Functioning			
A. Appears anxious or fearful of new people, situations			
B. Needs total control of the environment—"runs the show"			

continued

076-1643753-5

Infant/Toddler Symptom Checklist:
25 to 30 Months (continued)

How concerned are you about the symptoms checked above? (Circle one.)

Not concerned   Slightly concerned   Moderately concerned   Very concerned

---

Comments:

Infant/Toddler Symptom Checklist: 25 to 30 Months

Name______________________________ Date______________

	Never or Sometimes	Most Times	Past
1. Self-Regulation			
A. Is frequently irritable, fussy			
B. Goes easily from whimper to intense cry			
C. Can't calm self effectively by sucking on pacifier, looking at toys, or listening to caregiver			
D. Is unable to wait for food or toy without falling apart			
E. Can't change from one activity to another without distress (Must be prepared several times in advance before change is introduced)			
F. Amount of time spent calming child during day (circle one): 15-30 minutes 1-2 hours 3 hours +			
2. Attention			
A. Is easily distractible, has fleeting attention			
B. Tunes out from activity, is difficult to reengage			
C. Can't shift focus easily from one object or activity to another			
3. Sleep			
Requires extensive help to fall asleep; *specify:* rocking, long walks, stroking hair, car ride, other: ______________			
4. Dressing, Bathing, Touch			
Is distressed when face or hair washed			
5. Movement			
A. Is in constant movement, rocking, running about, unable to sit still for an activity			
B. Is fearful of being swung in air, swings, merry-go-rounds			
6. Looking and Sight			
A. Is sensitive to bright lights—cries or closes eyes			
B. Becomes excited in crowded, bustling settings such as supermarkets, restaurants			
7. Attachment/Emotional Functioning			
A. Appears anxious or fearful of new people, situations			
B. Needs total control of the environment—"runs the show"			

continued

076-1643753-5

Infant/Toddler Symptom Checklist:
25 to 30 Months (continued)

How concerned are you about the symptoms checked above? (Circle one.)

Not concerned   Slightly concerned   Moderately concerned   Very concerned

---

Comments:

Infant/Toddler Symptom Checklist:
25 to 30 Months

Name______________________________ Date______________

	Never or Sometimes	Most Times	Past
1. Self-Regulation			
A. Is frequently irritable, fussy			
B. Goes easily from whimper to intense cry			
C. Can't calm self effectively by sucking on pacifier, looking at toys, or listening to caregiver			
D. Is unable to wait for food or toy without falling apart			
E. Can't change from one activity to another without distress (Must be prepared several times in advance before change is introduced)			
F. Amount of time spent calming child during day (circle one): 15-30 minutes 1-2 hours 3 hours +			
2. Attention			
A. Is easily distractible, has fleeting attention			
B. Tunes out from activity, is difficult to reengage			
C. Can't shift focus easily from one object or activity to another			
3. Sleep			
Requires extensive help to fall asleep; *specify:* rocking, long walks, stroking hair, car ride, other: ______________			
4. Dressing, Bathing, Touch			
Is distressed when face or hair washed			
5. Movement			
A. Is in constant movement, rocking, running about, unable to sit still for an activity			
B. Is fearful of being swung in air, swings, merry-go-rounds			
6. Looking and Sight			
A. Is sensitive to bright lights—cries or closes eyes			
B. Becomes excited in crowded, bustling settings such as supermarkets, restaurants			
7. Attachment/Emotional Functioning			
A. Appears anxious or fearful of new people, situations			
B. Needs total control of the environment—"runs the show"			

continued

Infant/Toddler Symptom Checklist:
25 to 30 Months (continued)

How concerned are you about the symptoms checked above? (Circle one.)

Not concerned   Slightly concerned   Moderately concerned   Very concerned

---

Comments:

Infant/Toddler Symptom Checklist: 25 to 30 Months

Name______________________________ Date______________

	Never or Sometimes	Most Times	Past
1. Self-Regulation			
A. Is frequently irritable, fussy			
B. Goes easily from whimper to intense cry			
C. Can't calm self effectively by sucking on pacifier, looking at toys, or listening to caregiver			
D. Is unable to wait for food or toy without falling apart			
E. Can't change from one activity to another without distress (Must be prepared several times in advance before change is introduced)			
F. Amount of time spent calming child during day (circle one): 15-30 minutes 1-2 hours 3 hours +			
2. Attention			
A. Is easily distractible, has fleeting attention			
B. Tunes out from activity, is difficult to reengage			
C. Can't shift focus easily from one object or activity to another			
3. Sleep			
Requires extensive help to fall asleep; *specify:* rocking, long walks, stroking hair, car ride, other: ______________			
4. Dressing, Bathing, Touch			
Is distressed when face or hair washed			
5. Movement			
A. Is in constant movement, rocking, running about, unable to sit still for an activity			
B. Is fearful of being swung in air, swings, merry-go-rounds			
6. Looking and Sight			
A. Is sensitive to bright lights—cries or closes eyes			
B. Becomes excited in crowded, bustling settings such as supermarkets, restaurants			
7. Attachment/Emotional Functioning			
A. Appears anxious or fearful of new people, situations			
B. Needs total control of the environment—"runs the show"			

continued

076-1643753-5

Infant/Toddler Symptom Checklist:
25 to 30 Months (continued)

How concerned are you about the symptoms checked above? (Circle one.)

Not concerned Slightly concerned Moderately concerned Very concerned

Comments:

Infant/Toddler Symptom Checklist:
General Screening Version

Name________________________ Date____________

	Never or Sometimes	Most Times	Past
1. Is frequently irritable, fussy			
2. Goes easily from whimper to intense cry			
3. Can't calm self effectively by sucking on pacifier, looking at toys, or listening to caregiver			
4. Is unable to wait for food or toy without falling apart			
5. Demands adult company constantly			
6. Amount of time spent calming child during day (circle one): 15-30 minutes 1-2 hours 3 hours +			
7. Is easily distracted, has fleeting attention (for infants more than 1 year old)			
8. Wakes 3 or more times in the night and is unable to fall back to sleep			
9. Requires extensive help to fall asleep; *specify:* rocking, long walking, stroking hair, car ride, other: ____________			
10. Is distressed by having face or hair washed			
11. Resists cuddling; pulls away or arches			
12. Resists being placed in certain positions, such as on stomach, back			
13. Is in constant movement, rocking, running about; is unable to sit still for an activity			
14. Craves swinging and moving upside-down			
15. Startles or is distressed by loud sounds, such as vacuum, doorbell, or barking dog			
16. Is sensitive to bright lights—cries or closes eyes			
17. Becomes excited in crowded, bustling settings such as supermarkets, restaurants			
18. Has difficulty separating from parents, school, or babysitter			
19. Does not respond at all to limits, discipline			
20. Appears anxious or fearful of new people, situations			
21. Needs total control of the environment—"runs the show"			

How concerned are you about the symptoms checked above? (Circle one.)

Not concerned   Slightly concerned   Moderately concerned   Very concerned

continued

076-1643753-6

Infant/Toddler Symptom Checklist:
General Screening Version (continued)

Comments:

Infant/Toddler Symptom Checklist:
General Screening Version

Name____ Date_______________

	Never or Sometimes	Most Times	Past
1. Is frequently irritable, fussy			
2. Goes easily from whimper to intense cry			
3. Can't calm self effectively by sucking on pacifier, looking at toys, or listening to caregiver			
4. Is unable to wait for food or toy without falling apart			
5. Demands adult company constantly			
6. Amount of time spent calming child during day (circle one): 15-30 minutes 1-2 hours 3 hours +			
7. Is easily distracted, has fleeting attention (for infants more than 1 year old)			
8. Wakes 3 or more times in the night and is unable to fall back to sleep			
9. Requires extensive help to fall asleep; *specify:* rocking, long walking, stroking hair, car ride, other: ______________________			
10. Is distressed by having face or hair washed			
11. Resists cuddling; pulls away or arches			
12. Resists being placed in certain positions, such as on stomach, back			
13. Is in constant movement, rocking, running about; is unable to sit still for an activity			
14. Craves swinging and moving upside-down			
15. Startles or is distressed by loud sounds, such as vacuum, doorbell, or barking dog			
16. Is sensitive to bright lights—cries or closes eyes			
17. Becomes excited in crowded, bustling settings such as supermarkets, restaurants			
18. Has difficulty separating from parents, school, or babysitter			
19. Does not respond at all to limits, discipline			
20. Appears anxious or fearful of new people, situations			
21. Needs total control of the environment—"runs the show"			

How concerned are you about the symptoms checked above? (Circle one.)

Not concerned   Slightly concerned   Moderately concerned   Very concerned

continued

076-1643753-6

Infant/Toddler Symptom Checklist:
General Screening Version (continued)

Comments:

Infant/Toddler Symptom Checklist:
General Screening Version

Name______________________ Date__________

	Never or Sometimes	Most Times	Past
1. Is frequently irritable, fussy			
2. Goes easily from whimper to intense cry			
3. Can't calm self effectively by sucking on pacifier, looking at toys, or listening to caregiver			
4. Is unable to wait for food or toy without falling apart			
5. Demands adult company constantly			

6. Amount of time spent calming child during day (circle one):

15-30 minutes 1-2 hours 3 hours +

7. Is easily distracted, has fleeting attention (for infants more than 1 year old)			
8. Wakes 3 or more times in the night and is unable to fall back to sleep			
9. Requires extensive help to fall asleep; *specify:* rocking, long walking, stroking hair, car ride, other: ______________			
10. Is distressed by having face or hair washed			
11. Resists cuddling; pulls away or arches			
12. Resists being placed in certain positions, such as on stomach, back			
13. Is in constant movement, rocking, running about; is unable to sit still for an activity			
14. Craves swinging and moving upside-down			
15. Startles or is distressed by loud sounds, such as vacuum, doorbell, or barking dog			
16. Is sensitive to bright lights—cries or closes eyes			
17. Becomes excited in crowded, bustling settings such as supermarkets, restaurants			
18. Has difficulty separating from parents, school, or babysitter			
19. Does not respond at all to limits, discipline			
20. Appears anxious or fearful of new people, situations			
21. Needs total control of the environment—"runs the show"			

How concerned are you about the symptoms checked above? (Circle one.)

Not concerned Slightly concerned Moderately concerned Very concerned

continued

076-1643753-6

Infant/Toddler Symptom Checklist:
General Screening Version (continued)

Comments:

Infant/Toddler Symptom Checklist:
General Screening Version

Name____ Date________________

	Never or Sometimes	Most Times	Past
1. Is frequently irritable, fussy			
2. Goes easily from whimper to intense cry			
3. Can't calm self effectively by sucking on pacifier, looking at toys, or listening to caregiver			
4. Is unable to wait for food or toy without falling apart			
5. Demands adult company constantly			
6. Amount of time spent calming child during day (circle one): 15-30 minutes 1-2 hours 3 hours +			
7. Is easily distracted, has fleeting attention (for infants more than 1 year old)			
8. Wakes 3 or more times in the night and is unable to fall back to sleep			
9. Requires extensive help to fall asleep; *specify:* rocking, long walking, stroking hair, car ride, other: ____________________			
10. Is distressed by having face or hair washed			
11. Resists cuddling; pulls away or arches			
12. Resists being placed in certain positions, such as on stomach, back			
13. Is in constant movement, rocking, running about; is unable to sit still for an activity			
14. Craves swinging and moving upside-down			
15. Startles or is distressed by loud sounds, such as vacuum, doorbell, or barking dog			
16. Is sensitive to bright lights—cries or closes eyes			
17. Becomes excited in crowded, bustling settings such as supermarkets, restaurants			
18. Has difficulty separating from parents, school, or babysitter			
19. Does not respond at all to limits, discipline			
20. Appears anxious or fearful of new people, situations			
21. Needs total control of the environment—"runs the show"			

How concerned are you about the symptoms checked above? (Circle one.)

Not concerned Slightly concerned Moderately concerned Very concerned

continued

076-1643753-6

Infant/Toddler Symptom Checklist:
General Screening Version (continued)

Comments:

Infant/Toddler Symptom Checklist:
General Screening Version

Name__________________________________ Date____________

	Never or Sometimes	Most Times	Past
1. Is frequently irritable, fussy			
2. Goes easily from whimper to intense cry			
3. Can't calm self effectively by sucking on pacifier, looking at toys, or listening to caregiver			
4. Is unable to wait for food or toy without falling apart			
5. Demands adult company constantly			
6. Amount of time spent calming child during day (circle one): 15-30 minutes 1-2 hours 3 hours +			
7. Is easily distracted, has fleeting attention (for infants more than 1 year old)			
8. Wakes 3 or more times in the night and is unable to fall back to sleep			
9. Requires extensive help to fall asleep; *specify:* rocking, long walking, stroking hair, car ride, other: ____________			
10. Is distressed by having face or hair washed			
11. Resists cuddling; pulls away or arches			
12. Resists being placed in certain positions, such as on stomach, back			
13. Is in constant movement, rocking, running about; is unable to sit still for an activity			
14. Craves swinging and moving upside-down			
15. Startles or is distressed by loud sounds, such as vacuum, doorbell, or barking dog			
16. Is sensitive to bright lights—cries or closes eyes			
17. Becomes excited in crowded, bustling settings such as supermarkets, restaurants			
18. Has difficulty separating from parents, school, or babysitter			
19. Does not respond at all to limits, discipline			
20. Appears anxious or fearful of new people, situations			
21. Needs total control of the environment—"runs the show"			

How concerned are you about the symptoms checked above? (Circle one.)

Not concerned   Slightly concerned   Moderately concerned   Very concerned

continued

076-1643753-6

Infant/Toddler Symptom Checklist:
General Screening Version (continued)

Comments:

Infant/Toddler Symptom Checklist:
General Screening Version

Name____________________________________ Date______________

	Never or Sometimes	Most Times	Past
1. Is frequently irritable, fussy			
2. Goes easily from whimper to intense cry			
3. Can't calm self effectively by sucking on pacifier, looking at toys, or listening to caregiver			
4. Is unable to wait for food or toy without falling apart			
5. Demands adult company constantly			
6. Amount of time spent calming child during day (circle one): 15-30 minutes 1-2 hours 3 hours +			
7. Is easily distracted, has fleeting attention (for infants more than 1 year old)			
8. Wakes 3 or more times in the night and is unable to fall back to sleep			
9. Requires extensive help to fall asleep; *specify:* rocking, long walking, stroking hair, car ride, other: ________________			
10. Is distressed by having face or hair washed			
11. Resists cuddling; pulls away or arches			
12. Resists being placed in certain positions, such as on stomach, back			
13. Is in constant movement, rocking, running about; is unable to sit still for an activity			
14. Craves swinging and moving upside-down			
15. Startles or is distressed by loud sounds, such as vacuum, doorbell, or barking dog			
16. Is sensitive to bright lights—cries or closes eyes			
17. Becomes excited in crowded, bustling settings such as supermarkets, restaurants			
18. Has difficulty separating from parents, school, or babysitter			
19. Does not respond at all to limits, discipline			
20. Appears anxious or fearful of new people, situations			
21. Needs total control of the environment—"runs the show"			

How concerned are you about the symptoms checked above? (Circle one.)

Not concerned Slightly concerned Moderately concerned Very concerned

continued

076-1643753-6

Infant/Toddler Symptom Checklist:
General Screening Version (continued)

Comments:

Infant/Toddler Symptom Checklist:
General Screening Version

Name________________________ Date____________

	Never or Sometimes	Most Times	Past
1. Is frequently irritable, fussy			
2. Goes easily from whimper to intense cry			
3. Can't calm self effectively by sucking on pacifier, looking at toys, or listening to caregiver			
4. Is unable to wait for food or toy without falling apart			
5. Demands adult company constantly			
6. Amount of time spent calming child during day (circle one): 15-30 minutes 1-2 hours 3 hours +			
7. Is easily distracted, has fleeting attention (for infants more than 1 year old)			
8. Wakes 3 or more times in the night and is unable to fall back to sleep			
9. Requires extensive help to fall asleep; *specify:* rocking, long walking, stroking hair, car ride, other: ____________			
10. Is distressed by having face or hair washed			
11. Resists cuddling; pulls away or arches			
12. Resists being placed in certain positions, such as on stomach, back			
13. Is in constant movement, rocking, running about; is unable to sit still for an activity			
14. Craves swinging and moving upside-down			
15. Startles or is distressed by loud sounds, such as vacuum, doorbell, or barking dog			
16. Is sensitive to bright lights—cries or closes eyes			
17. Becomes excited in crowded, bustling settings such as supermarkets, restaurants			
18. Has difficulty separating from parents, school, or babysitter			
19. Does not respond at all to limits, discipline			
20. Appears anxious or fearful of new people, situations			
21. Needs total control of the environment—"runs the show"			

How concerned are you about the symptoms checked above? (Circle one.)

Not concerned Slightly concerned Moderately concerned Very concerned

continued

076-1643753-6

Infant/Toddler Symptom Checklist:
General Screening Version (continued)

Comments:

Infant/Toddler Symptom Checklist:
General Screening Version

Name____ Date________________

		Never or Sometimes	Most Times	Past
1.	Is frequently irritable, fussy			
2.	Goes easily from whimper to intense cry			
3.	Can't calm self effectively by sucking on pacifier, looking at toys, or listening to caregiver			
4.	Is unable to wait for food or toy without falling apart			
5.	Demands adult company constantly			
6.	Amount of time spent calming child during day (circle one): 15-30 minutes 1-2 hours 3 hours +			
7.	Is easily distracted, has fleeting attention (for infants more than 1 year old)			
8.	Wakes 3 or more times in the night and is unable to fall back to sleep			
9.	Requires extensive help to fall asleep; *specify:* rocking, long walking, stroking hair, car ride, other: ____________________			
10.	Is distressed by having face or hair washed			
11.	Resists cuddling; pulls away or arches			
12.	Resists being placed in certain positions, such as on stomach, back			
13.	Is in constant movement, rocking, running about; is unable to sit still for an activity			
14.	Craves swinging and moving upside-down			
15.	Startles or is distressed by loud sounds, such as vacuum, doorbell, or barking dog			
16.	Is sensitive to bright lights—cries or closes eyes			
17.	Becomes excited in crowded, bustling settings such as supermarkets, restaurants			
18.	Has difficulty separating from parents, school, or babysitter			
19.	Does not respond at all to limits, discipline			
20.	Appears anxious or fearful of new people, situations			
21.	Needs total control of the environment—"runs the show"			

How concerned are you about the symptoms checked above? (Circle one.)

Not concerned   Slightly concerned   Moderately concerned   Very concerned

continued

076-1643753-6

Comments:

Infant/Toddler Symptom Checklist:
General Screening Version

Name______________________________ Date______________

	Never or Sometimes	Most Times	Past
1. Is frequently irritable, fussy			
2. Goes easily from whimper to intense cry			
3. Can't calm self effectively by sucking on pacifier, looking at toys, or listening to caregiver			
4. Is unable to wait for food or toy without falling apart			
5. Demands adult company constantly			
6. Amount of time spent calming child during day (circle one): 15-30 minutes 1-2 hours 3 hours +			
7. Is easily distracted, has fleeting attention (for infants more than 1 year old)			
8. Wakes 3 or more times in the night and is unable to fall back to sleep			
9. Requires extensive help to fall asleep; *specify:* rocking, long walking, stroking hair, car ride, other: ____________			
10. Is distressed by having face or hair washed			
11. Resists cuddling; pulls away or arches			
12. Resists being placed in certain positions, such as on stomach, back			
13. Is in constant movement, rocking, running about; is unable to sit still for an activity			
14. Craves swinging and moving upside-down			
15. Startles or is distressed by loud sounds, such as vacuum, doorbell, or barking dog			
16. Is sensitive to bright lights—cries or closes eyes			
17. Becomes excited in crowded, bustling settings such as supermarkets, restaurants			
18. Has difficulty separating from parents, school, or babysitter			
19. Does not respond at all to limits, discipline			
20. Appears anxious or fearful of new people, situations			
21. Needs total control of the environment—"runs the show"			

How concerned are you about the symptoms checked above? (Circle one.)

Not concerned   Slightly concerned   Moderately concerned   Very concerned

continued

076-1643753-6

Infant/Toddler Symptom Checklist:
General Screening Version (continued)

Comments:

Infant/Toddler Symptom Checklist:
General Screening Version

Name____ Date______________

	Never or Sometimes	Most Times	Past
1. Is frequently irritable, fussy			
2. Goes easily from whimper to intense cry			
3. Can't calm self effectively by sucking on pacifier, looking at toys, or listening to caregiver			
4. Is unable to wait for food or toy without falling apart			
5. Demands adult company constantly			
6. Amount of time spent calming child during day (circle one): 15-30 minutes 1-2 hours 3 hours +			
7. Is easily distracted, has fleeting attention (for infants more than 1 year old)			
8. Wakes 3 or more times in the night and is unable to fall back to sleep			
9. Requires extensive help to fall asleep; *specify:* rocking, long walking, stroking hair, car ride, other: ____________________			
10. Is distressed by having face or hair washed			
11. Resists cuddling; pulls away or arches			
12. Resists being placed in certain positions, such as on stomach, back			
13. Is in constant movement, rocking, running about; is unable to sit still for an activity			
14. Craves swinging and moving upside-down			
15. Startles or is distressed by loud sounds, such as vacuum, doorbell, or barking dog			
16. Is sensitive to bright lights—cries or closes eyes			
17. Becomes excited in crowded, bustling settings such as supermarkets, restaurants			
18. Has difficulty separating from parents, school, or babysitter			
19. Does not respond at all to limits, discipline			
20. Appears anxious or fearful of new people, situations			
21. Needs total control of the environment—"runs the show"			

How concerned are you about the symptoms checked above? (Circle one.)

Not concerned   Slightly concerned   Moderately concerned   Very concerned

continued

076-1643753-6

Infant/Toddler Symptom Checklist:
General Screening Version (continued)

Comments:

Infant/Toddler Symptom Checklist:
General Screening Version

Name______________________________ Date______________

	Never or Sometimes	Most Times	Past
1. Is frequently irritable, fussy			
2. Goes easily from whimper to intense cry			
3. Can't calm self effectively by sucking on pacifier, looking at toys, or listening to caregiver			
4. Is unable to wait for food or toy without falling apart			
5. Demands adult company constantly			
6. Amount of time spent calming child during day (circle one): 15-30 minutes 1-2 hours 3 hours +			
7. Is easily distracted, has fleeting attention (for infants more than 1 year old)			
8. Wakes 3 or more times in the night and is unable to fall back to sleep			
9. Requires extensive help to fall asleep; *specify:* rocking, long walking, stroking hair, car ride, other: ______________			
10. Is distressed by having face or hair washed			
11. Resists cuddling; pulls away or arches			
12. Resists being placed in certain positions, such as on stomach, back			
13. Is in constant movement, rocking, running about; is unable to sit still for an activity			
14. Craves swinging and moving upside-down			
15. Startles or is distressed by loud sounds, such as vacuum, doorbell, or barking dog			
16. Is sensitive to bright lights—cries or closes eyes			
17. Becomes excited in crowded, bustling settings such as supermarkets, restaurants			
18. Has difficulty separating from parents, school, or babysitter			
19. Does not respond at all to limits, discipline			
20. Appears anxious or fearful of new people, situations			
21. Needs total control of the environment—"runs the show"			

How concerned are you about the symptoms checked above? (Circle one.)

Not concerned Slightly concerned Moderately concerned Very concerned

continued

076-1643753-6

Infant/Toddler Symptom Checklist:
General Screening Version (continued)

Comments:

Infant/Toddler Symptom Checklist:
General Screening Version

Name________________________________ Date________________

	Never or Sometimes	Most Times	Past
1. Is frequently irritable, fussy			
2. Goes easily from whimper to intense cry			
3. Can't calm self effectively by sucking on pacifier, looking at toys, or listening to caregiver			
4. Is unable to wait for food or toy without falling apart			
5. Demands adult company constantly			
6. Amount of time spent calming child during day (circle one): 15-30 minutes 1-2 hours 3 hours +			
7. Is easily distracted, has fleeting attention (for infants more than 1 year old)			
8. Wakes 3 or more times in the night and is unable to fall back to sleep			
9. Requires extensive help to fall asleep; *specify:* rocking, long walking, stroking hair, car ride, other: ________________			
10. Is distressed by having face or hair washed			
11. Resists cuddling; pulls away or arches			
12. Resists being placed in certain positions, such as on stomach, back			
13. Is in constant movement, rocking, running about; is unable to sit still for an activity			
14. Craves swinging and moving upside-down			
15. Startles or is distressed by loud sounds, such as vacuum, doorbell, or barking dog			
16. Is sensitive to bright lights—cries or closes eyes			
17. Becomes excited in crowded, bustling settings such as supermarkets, restaurants			
18. Has difficulty separating from parents, school, or babysitter			
19. Does not respond at all to limits, discipline			
20. Appears anxious or fearful of new people, situations			
21. Needs total control of the environment—"runs the show"			

How concerned are you about the symptoms checked above? (Circle one.)

Not concerned   Slightly concerned   Moderately concerned   Very concerned

continued

076-1643753-6

Infant/Toddler Symptom Checklist:
General Screening Version (continued)

Comments:

Infant/Toddler Symptom Checklist:
General Screening Version

Name______________________________ Date______________

		Never or Sometimes	Most Times	Past
1.	Is frequently irritable, fussy			
2.	Goes easily from whimper to intense cry			
3.	Can't calm self effectively by sucking on pacifier, looking at toys, or listening to caregiver			
4.	Is unable to wait for food or toy without falling apart			
5.	Demands adult company constantly			
6.	Amount of time spent calming child during day (circle one): 15-30 minutes 1-2 hours 3 hours +			
7.	Is easily distracted, has fleeting attention (for infants more than 1 year old)			
8.	Wakes 3 or more times in the night and is unable to fall back to sleep			
9.	Requires extensive help to fall asleep; *specify:* rocking, long walking, stroking hair, car ride, other: ____________			
10.	Is distressed by having face or hair washed			
11.	Resists cuddling; pulls away or arches			
12.	Resists being placed in certain positions, such as on stomach, back			
13.	Is in constant movement, rocking, running about; is unable to sit still for an activity			
14.	Craves swinging and moving upside-down			
15.	Startles or is distressed by loud sounds, such as vacuum, doorbell, or barking dog			
16.	Is sensitive to bright lights—cries or closes eyes			
17.	Becomes excited in crowded, bustling settings such as supermarkets, restaurants			
18.	Has difficulty separating from parents, school, or babysitter			
19.	Does not respond at all to limits, discipline			
20.	Appears anxious or fearful of new people, situations			
21.	Needs total control of the environment—"runs the show"			

How concerned are you about the symptoms checked above? (Circle one.)

Not concerned   Slightly concerned   Moderately concerned   Very concerned

continued

076-1643753-6

Infant/Toddler Symptom Checklist:
General Screening Version (continued)

Comments:

Infant/Toddler Symptom Checklist:
General Screening Version

Name_______________________________ Date____________

		Never or Sometimes	Most Times	Past
1.	Is frequently irritable, fussy			
2.	Goes easily from whimper to intense cry			
3.	Can't calm self effectively by sucking on pacifier, looking at toys, or listening to caregiver			
4.	Is unable to wait for food or toy without falling apart			
5.	Demands adult company constantly			
6.	Amount of time spent calming child during day (circle one): 15-30 minutes 1-2 hours 3 hours +			
7.	Is easily distracted, has fleeting attention (for infants more than 1 year old)			
8.	Wakes 3 or more times in the night and is unable to fall back to sleep			
9.	Requires extensive help to fall asleep; *specify:* rocking, long walking, stroking hair, car ride, other: ______________			
10.	Is distressed by having face or hair washed			
11.	Resists cuddling; pulls away or arches			
12.	Resists being placed in certain positions, such as on stomach, back			
13.	Is in constant movement, rocking, running about; is unable to sit still for an activity			
14.	Craves swinging and moving upside-down			
15.	Startles or is distressed by loud sounds, such as vacuum, doorbell, or barking dog			
16.	Is sensitive to bright lights—cries or closes eyes			
17.	Becomes excited in crowded, bustling settings such as supermarkets, restaurants			
18.	Has difficulty separating from parents, school, or babysitter			
19.	Does not respond at all to limits, discipline			
20.	Appears anxious or fearful of new people, situations			
21.	Needs total control of the environment—"runs the show"			

How concerned are you about the symptoms checked above? (Circle one.)

Not concerned Slightly concerned Moderately concerned Very concerned

continued

076-1643753-6

Infant/Toddler Symptom Checklist:
General Screening Version (continued)

Comments:

Infant/Toddler Symptom Checklist:
General Screening Version

Name____ Date______________

		Never or Sometimes	Most Times	Past
1.	Is frequently irritable, fussy			
2.	Goes easily from whimper to intense cry			
3.	Can't calm self effectively by sucking on pacifier, looking at toys, or listening to caregiver			
4.	Is unable to wait for food or toy without falling apart			
5.	Demands adult company constantly			
6.	Amount of time spent calming child during day (circle one): 15-30 minutes 1-2 hours 3 hours +			
7.	Is easily distracted, has fleeting attention (for infants more than 1 year old)			
8.	Wakes 3 or more times in the night and is unable to fall back to sleep			
9.	Requires extensive help to fall asleep; *specify:* rocking, long walking, stroking hair, car ride, other: ______________________			
10.	Is distressed by having face or hair washed			
11.	Resists cuddling; pulls away or arches			
12.	Resists being placed in certain positions, such as on stomach, back			
13.	Is in constant movement, rocking, running about; is unable to sit still for an activity			
14.	Craves swinging and moving upside-down			
15.	Startles or is distressed by loud sounds, such as vacuum, doorbell, or barking dog			
16.	Is sensitive to bright lights—cries or closes eyes			
17.	Becomes excited in crowded, bustling settings such as supermarkets, restaurants			
18.	Has difficulty separating from parents, school, or babysitter			
19.	Does not respond at all to limits, discipline			
20.	Appears anxious or fearful of new people, situations			
21.	Needs total control of the environment—"runs the show"			

How concerned are you about the symptoms checked above? (Circle one.)

Not concerned   Slightly concerned   Moderately concerned   Very concerned

continued

076-1643753-6

Infant/Toddler Symptom Checklist:
General Screening Version (continued)

Comments:

Infant/Toddler Symptom Checklist:
General Screening Version

Name____ Date_______________

		Never or Sometimes	Most Times	Past
1.	Is frequently irritable, fussy			
2.	Goes easily from whimper to intense cry			
3.	Can't calm self effectively by sucking on pacifier, looking at toys, or listening to caregiver			
4.	Is unable to wait for food or toy without falling apart			
5.	Demands adult company constantly			
6.	Amount of time spent calming child during day (circle one): 15-30 minutes 1-2 hours 3 hours +			
7.	Is easily distracted, has fleeting attention (for infants more than 1 year old)			
8.	Wakes 3 or more times in the night and is unable to fall back to sleep			
9.	Requires extensive help to fall asleep; *specify:* rocking, long walking, stroking hair, car ride, other: ______________________			
10.	Is distressed by having face or hair washed			
11.	Resists cuddling; pulls away or arches			
12.	Resists being placed in certain positions, such as on stomach, back			
13.	Is in constant movement, rocking, running about; is unable to sit still for an activity			
14.	Craves swinging and moving upside-down			
15.	Startles or is distressed by loud sounds, such as vacuum, doorbell, or barking dog			
16.	Is sensitive to bright lights—cries or closes eyes			
17.	Becomes excited in crowded, bustling settings such as supermarkets, restaurants			
18.	Has difficulty separating from parents, school, or babysitter			
19.	Does not respond at all to limits, discipline			
20.	Appears anxious or fearful of new people, situations			
21.	Needs total control of the environment—"runs the show"			

How concerned are you about the symptoms checked above? (Circle one.)

Not concerned Slightly concerned Moderately concerned Very concerned

continued

076-1643753-6

Infant/Toddler Symptom Checklist:
General Screening Version (continued)

Comments:

Infant/Toddler Symptom Checklist:
General Screening Version

Name______________________________ Date______________

	Never or Sometimes	Most Times	Past
1. Is frequently irritable, fussy			
2. Goes easily from whimper to intense cry			
3. Can't calm self effectively by sucking on pacifier, looking at toys, or listening to caregiver			
4. Is unable to wait for food or toy without falling apart			
5. Demands adult company constantly			
6. Amount of time spent calming child during day (circle one): 15-30 minutes 1-2 hours 3 hours +			
7. Is easily distracted, has fleeting attention (for infants more than 1 year old)			
8. Wakes 3 or more times in the night and is unable to fall back to sleep			
9. Requires extensive help to fall asleep; *specify:* rocking, long walking, stroking hair, car ride, other: ______________			
10. Is distressed by having face or hair washed			
11. Resists cuddling; pulls away or arches			
12. Resists being placed in certain positions, such as on stomach, back			
13. Is in constant movement, rocking, running about; is unable to sit still for an activity			
14. Craves swinging and moving upside-down			
15. Startles or is distressed by loud sounds, such as vacuum, doorbell, or barking dog			
16. Is sensitive to bright lights—cries or closes eyes			
17. Becomes excited in crowded, bustling settings such as supermarkets, restaurants			
18. Has difficulty separating from parents, school, or babysitter			
19. Does not respond at all to limits, discipline			
20. Appears anxious or fearful of new people, situations			
21. Needs total control of the environment—"runs the show"			

How concerned are you about the symptoms checked above? (Circle one.)

Not concerned   Slightly concerned   Moderately concerned   Very concerned

continued

076-1643753-6

Infant/Toddler Symptom Checklist:
General Screening Version (continued)

Comments:

Infant/Toddler Symptom Checklist:
General Screening Version

Name______________________________ Date______________

	Never or Sometimes	Most Times	Past
1. Is frequently irritable, fussy			
2. Goes easily from whimper to intense cry			
3. Can't calm self effectively by sucking on pacifier, looking at toys, or listening to caregiver			
4. Is unable to wait for food or toy without falling apart			
5. Demands adult company constantly			
6. Amount of time spent calming child during day (circle one): 15-30 minutes 1-2 hours 3 hours +			
7. Is easily distracted, has fleeting attention (for infants more than 1 year old)			
8. Wakes 3 or more times in the night and is unable to fall back to sleep			
9. Requires extensive help to fall asleep; *specify*: rocking, long walking, stroking hair, car ride, other: ____________			
10. Is distressed by having face or hair washed			
11. Resists cuddling; pulls away or arches			
12. Resists being placed in certain positions, such as on stomach, back			
13. Is in constant movement, rocking, running about; is unable to sit still for an activity			
14. Craves swinging and moving upside-down			
15. Startles or is distressed by loud sounds, such as vacuum, doorbell, or barking dog			
16. Is sensitive to bright lights—cries or closes eyes			
17. Becomes excited in crowded, bustling settings such as supermarkets, restaurants			
18. Has difficulty separating from parents, school, or babysitter			
19. Does not respond at all to limits, discipline			
20. Appears anxious or fearful of new people, situations			
21. Needs total control of the environment—"runs the show"			

How concerned are you about the symptoms checked above? (Circle one.)

Not concerned   Slightly concerned   Moderately concerned   Very concerned

continued

076-1643753-6

Infant/Toddler Symptom Checklist:
General Screening Version (continued)

Comments:

Infant/Toddler Symptom Checklist:
General Screening Version

Name______________________________ Date______________

	Never or Sometimes	Most Times	Past
1. Is frequently irritable, fussy			
2. Goes easily from whimper to intense cry			
3. Can't calm self effectively by sucking on pacifier, looking at toys, or listening to caregiver			
4. Is unable to wait for food or toy without falling apart			
5. Demands adult company constantly			

6. Amount of time spent calming child during day (circle one):

15-30 minutes   1-2 hours   3 hours +

7. Is easily distracted, has fleeting attention (for infants more than 1 year old)			
8. Wakes 3 or more times in the night and is unable to fall back to sleep			
9. Requires extensive help to fall asleep; *specify:* rocking, long walking, stroking hair, car ride, other: ______________			
10. Is distressed by having face or hair washed			
11. Resists cuddling; pulls away or arches			
12. Resists being placed in certain positions, such as on stomach, back			
13. Is in constant movement, rocking, running about; is unable to sit still for an activity			
14. Craves swinging and moving upside-down			
15. Startles or is distressed by loud sounds, such as vacuum, doorbell, or barking dog			
16. Is sensitive to bright lights—cries or closes eyes			
17. Becomes excited in crowded, bustling settings such as supermarkets, restaurants			
18. Has difficulty separating from parents, school, or babysitter			
19. Does not respond at all to limits, discipline			
20. Appears anxious or fearful of new people, situations			
21. Needs total control of the environment—"runs the show"			

How concerned are you about the symptoms checked above? (Circle one.)

Not concerned   Slightly concerned   Moderately concerned   Very concerned

continued

076-1643753-6

Infant/Toddler Symptom Checklist:
General Screening Version (continued)

Comments:

Infant/Toddler Symptom Checklist:
General Screening Version

Name________________________________ Date______________

	Never or Sometimes	Most Times	Past
1. Is frequently irritable, fussy			
2. Goes easily from whimper to intense cry			
3. Can't calm self effectively by sucking on pacifier, looking at toys, or listening to caregiver			
4. Is unable to wait for food or toy without falling apart			
5. Demands adult company constantly			
6. Amount of time spent calming child during day (circle one): 15-30 minutes 1-2 hours 3 hours +			
7. Is easily distracted, has fleeting attention (for infants more than 1 year old)			
8. Wakes 3 or more times in the night and is unable to fall back to sleep			
9. Requires extensive help to fall asleep; *specify:* rocking, long walking, stroking hair, car ride, other: ____________			
10. Is distressed by having face or hair washed			
11. Resists cuddling; pulls away or arches			
12. Resists being placed in certain positions, such as on stomach, back			
13. Is in constant movement, rocking, running about; is unable to sit still for an activity			
14. Craves swinging and moving upside-down			
15. Startles or is distressed by loud sounds, such as vacuum, doorbell, or barking dog			
16. Is sensitive to bright lights—cries or closes eyes			
17. Becomes excited in crowded, bustling settings such as supermarkets, restaurants			
18. Has difficulty separating from parents, school, or babysitter			
19. Does not respond at all to limits, discipline			
20. Appears anxious or fearful of new people, situations			
21. Needs total control of the environment—"runs the show"			

How concerned are you about the symptoms checked above? (Circle one.)

Not concerned   Slightly concerned   Moderately concerned   Very concerned

continued

076-1643753-6

Infant/Toddler Symptom Checklist:
General Screening Version (continued)

Comments:

Infant/Toddler Symptom Checklist:
General Screening Version

Name____________________ Date__________

	Never or Sometimes	Most Times	Past
1. Is frequently irritable, fussy			
2. Goes easily from whimper to intense cry			
3. Can't calm self effectively by sucking on pacifier, looking at toys, or listening to caregiver			
4. Is unable to wait for food or toy without falling apart			
5. Demands adult company constantly			
6. Amount of time spent calming child during day (circle one): 15-30 minutes 1-2 hours 3 hours +			
7. Is easily distracted, has fleeting attention (for infants more than 1 year old)			
8. Wakes 3 or more times in the night and is unable to fall back to sleep			
9. Requires extensive help to fall asleep; *specify:* rocking, long walking, stroking hair, car ride, other: ________			
10. Is distressed by having face or hair washed			
11. Resists cuddling; pulls away or arches			
12. Resists being placed in certain positions, such as on stomach, back			
13. Is in constant movement, rocking, running about; is unable to sit still for an activity			
14. Craves swinging and moving upside-down			
15. Startles or is distressed by loud sounds, such as vacuum, doorbell, or barking dog			
16. Is sensitive to bright lights—cries or closes eyes			
17. Becomes excited in crowded, bustling settings such as supermarkets, restaurants			
18. Has difficulty separating from parents, school, or babysitter			
19. Does not respond at all to limits, discipline			
20. Appears anxious or fearful of new people, situations			
21. Needs total control of the environment—"runs the show"			

How concerned are you about the symptoms checked above? (Circle one.)

Not concerned Slightly concerned Moderately concerned Very concerned

continued

076-1643753-6

Infant/Toddler Symptom Checklist:
General Screening Version (continued)

Comments:

Infant/Toddler Symptom Checklist:
General Screening Version

Name________________________________ Date____________

	Never or Sometimes	Most Times	Past
1. Is frequently irritable, fussy			
2. Goes easily from whimper to intense cry			
3. Can't calm self effectively by sucking on pacifier, looking at toys, or listening to caregiver			
4. Is unable to wait for food or toy without falling apart			
5. Demands adult company constantly			

6. Amount of time spent calming child during day (circle one):

15-30 minutes   1-2 hours   3 hours +

7. Is easily distracted, has fleeting attention (for infants more than 1 year old)			
8. Wakes 3 or more times in the night and is unable to fall back to sleep			
9. Requires extensive help to fall asleep; *specify:* rocking, long walking, stroking hair, car ride, other: ____________			
10. Is distressed by having face or hair washed			
11. Resists cuddling; pulls away or arches			
12. Resists being placed in certain positions, such as on stomach, back			
13. Is in constant movement, rocking, running about; is unable to sit still for an activity			
14. Craves swinging and moving upside-down			
15. Startles or is distressed by loud sounds, such as vacuum, doorbell, or barking dog			
16. Is sensitive to bright lights—cries or closes eyes			
17. Becomes excited in crowded, bustling settings such as supermarkets, restaurants			
18. Has difficulty separating from parents, school, or babysitter			
19. Does not respond at all to limits, discipline			
20. Appears anxious or fearful of new people, situations			
21. Needs total control of the environment—"runs the show"			

How concerned are you about the symptoms checked above? (Circle one.)

Not concerned   Slightly concerned   Moderately concerned   Very concerned

continued

076-1643753-6

Infant/Toddler Symptom Checklist:
General Screening Version (continued)

Comments:

Infant/Toddler Symptom Checklist:
General Screening Version

Name________________________________ Date______________

	Never or Sometimes	Most Times	Past
1. Is frequently irritable, fussy			
2. Goes easily from whimper to intense cry			
3. Can't calm self effectively by sucking on pacifier, looking at toys, or listening to caregiver			
4. Is unable to wait for food or toy without falling apart			
5. Demands adult company constantly			

6. Amount of time spent calming child during day (circle one):

15-30 minutes 1-2 hours 3 hours +

	Never or Sometimes	Most Times	Past
7. Is easily distracted, has fleeting attention (for infants more than 1 year old)			
8. Wakes 3 or more times in the night and is unable to fall back to sleep			
9. Requires extensive help to fall asleep; *specify:* rocking, long walking, stroking hair, car ride, other: ______________			
10. Is distressed by having face or hair washed			
11. Resists cuddling; pulls away or arches			
12. Resists being placed in certain positions, such as on stomach, back			
13. Is in constant movement, rocking, running about; is unable to sit still for an activity			
14. Craves swinging and moving upside-down			
15. Startles or is distressed by loud sounds, such as vacuum, doorbell, or barking dog			
16. Is sensitive to bright lights—cries or closes eyes			
17. Becomes excited in crowded, bustling settings such as supermarkets, restaurants			
18. Has difficulty separating from parents, school, or babysitter			
19. Does not respond at all to limits, discipline			
20. Appears anxious or fearful of new people, situations			
21. Needs total control of the environment—"runs the show"			

How concerned are you about the symptoms checked above? (Circle one.)

Not concerned Slightly concerned Moderately concerned Very concerned

continued

076-1643753-6

Comments:

Infant/Toddler Symptom Checklist:
General Screening Version

Name____________________________ Date____________

	Never or Sometimes	Most Times	Past
1. Is frequently irritable, fussy			
2. Goes easily from whimper to intense cry			
3. Can't calm self effectively by sucking on pacifier, looking at toys, or listening to caregiver			
4. Is unable to wait for food or toy without falling apart			
5. Demands adult company constantly			
6. Amount of time spent calming child during day (circle one): 15-30 minutes 1-2 hours 3 hours +			
7. Is easily distracted, has fleeting attention (for infants more than 1 year old)			
8. Wakes 3 or more times in the night and is unable to fall back to sleep			
9. Requires extensive help to fall asleep; *specify:* rocking, long walking, stroking hair, car ride, other: __________			
10. Is distressed by having face or hair washed			
11. Resists cuddling; pulls away or arches			
12. Resists being placed in certain positions, such as on stomach, back			
13. Is in constant movement, rocking, running about; is unable to sit still for an activity			
14. Craves swinging and moving upside-down			
15. Startles or is distressed by loud sounds, such as vacuum, doorbell, or barking dog			
16. Is sensitive to bright lights—cries or closes eyes			
17. Becomes excited in crowded, bustling settings such as supermarkets, restaurants			
18. Has difficulty separating from parents, school, or babysitter			
19. Does not respond at all to limits, discipline			
20. Appears anxious or fearful of new people, situations			
21. Needs total control of the environment—"runs the show"			

How concerned are you about the symptoms checked above? (Circle one.)

Not concerned Slightly concerned Moderately concerned Very concerned

continued

076-1643753-6

Infant/Toddler Symptom Checklist:
General Screening Version (continued)

Comments:

Infant/Toddler Symptom Checklist:
General Screening Version

Name____ Date______________

	Never or Sometimes	Most Times	Past
1. Is frequently irritable, fussy			
2. Goes easily from whimper to intense cry			
3. Can't calm self effectively by sucking on pacifier, looking at toys, or listening to caregiver			
4. Is unable to wait for food or toy without falling apart			
5. Demands adult company constantly			
6. Amount of time spent calming child during day (circle one): 15-30 minutes 1-2 hours 3 hours +			
7. Is easily distracted, has fleeting attention (for infants more than 1 year old)			
8. Wakes 3 or more times in the night and is unable to fall back to sleep			
9. Requires extensive help to fall asleep; *specify:* rocking, long walking, stroking hair, car ride, other: ______________________			
10. Is distressed by having face or hair washed			
11. Resists cuddling; pulls away or arches			
12. Resists being placed in certain positions, such as on stomach, back			
13. Is in constant movement, rocking, running about; is unable to sit still for an activity			
14. Craves swinging and moving upside-down			
15. Startles or is distressed by loud sounds, such as vacuum, doorbell, or barking dog			
16. Is sensitive to bright lights—cries or closes eyes			
17. Becomes excited in crowded, bustling settings such as supermarkets, restaurants			
18. Has difficulty separating from parents, school, or babysitter			
19. Does not respond at all to limits, discipline			
20. Appears anxious or fearful of new people, situations			
21. Needs total control of the environment—"runs the show"			

How concerned are you about the symptoms checked above? (Circle one.)

Not concerned Slightly concerned Moderately concerned Very concerned

continued

076-1643753-6

Infant/Toddler Symptom Checklist:
General Screening Version (continued)

Comments: